"Mounting evidence indicates that refined carbohydrates and high glycemic index foods are contributing to the escalating epidemics of obesity and type 2 diabetes worldwide. This dietary pattern also appears to increase the risk of heart disease and stroke. The skyrocketing proportion of calories from added sugars and refined carbohydrates in Westernized diets portends a future acceleration of these trends. *The Glucose Revolution* challenges traditional doctrines about optimal nutrition and the role of carbohydrates in health and disease. Brand-Miller and colleagues are to be congratulated for an eminently lucid and important book that explains the science behind the glycemic index and provides tools and strategies for modifying diet to incorporate this knowledge. I strongly recommend the book to both health professionals and the general public who could use this state-of-the-art information to improve health and well-being."

—JOANN E. MANSON, M.D., DR.P.H., Professor of Medicine, Harvard Medical School, and Co-Director of Women's Health, Division of Preventive Medicine, Brigham and Women's Hospital

■

"Here is at last a book explaining the importance of taking into consideration the glycemic index of foods for overall health, athletic performance, and in reducing the risk of heart disease and diabetes. The book clearly explains that there are different kinds of carbohydrates that work in different ways and why a universal recommendation to 'increase the carbohydrate content of your diet' is plainly simple and scientifically inaccurate. Everyone should put the glycemic index approach into practice."

—ARTEMIS P. SIMOPOULOS, M.D., senior author of
The Omega Diet and *The Healing Diet* and President,
The Center for Genetics, Nutrition and Health,
Washington, D.C., on *The Glucose Revolution*

"*The Glucose Revolution* is nutrition science for the 21st century. Clearly written, it gives the scientific rationale for why all carbohydrates are not created equal. It is a practical guide for both professionals and patients. The food suggestions and recipes are exciting and tasty."
—RICHARD N. PODELL, M.D., M.P.H., Clinical Professor, Department of Family Medicine, UMDNJ-Robert Wood Johnson Medical School, and co-author of *The G-Index Diet: The Missing Link That Makes Permanent Weight Loss Possible*

■

"The glycemic index is a useful tool which may have a broad spectrum of applications, from the maintenance of fuel supply during exercise to the control of blood glucose levels in diabetics. Low glycemic index foods may prove to have beneficial health effects for all of us in the long term. *The Glucose Revolution* is a user-friendly, easy-to-read overview of all that you need to know about the glycemic index. This book represents a balanced account of the importance of the glycemic index based on sound scientific evidence."
—JAMES HILL, PH.D., Director, Center for Human Nutrition, University of Colorado Health Sciences Center

■

"As a coach of elite amateur and professional athletes, I know how critical the glycemic index is to sports performance. *The New Glucose Revolution* provides the serious athlete with the basic tools necessary for getting the training table right."
—JOE FRIEL, coach, author, consultant

Other Glucose Revolution &
New Glucose Revolution Titles

*The New Glucose Revolution: The Authoritative Guide to the
Glycemic Index—the Dietary Solution for Lifelong Health*

The Low GI Diet Revolution

The Low GI Diet Cookbook

The New Glucose Revolution Life Plan

The New Glucose Revolution Low GI Eating Made Easy

*What Makes My Blood Glucose Go Up ... And Down?
And 101 Other Frequently Asked Questions
about Your Blood Glucose Levels*

*The New Glucose Revolution Complete Guide
to Glycemic Index Values*

The New Glucose Revolution Guide to Living Well with PCOS

■

*The New Glucose Revolution Pocket Guide to the
Top 100 Low GI Foods*

*The New Glucose Revolution Pocket Guide to
the Metabolic Syndrome and Your Heart*

The New Glucose Revolution Pocket Guide to Peak Performance

The New Glucose Revolution Pocket Guide to Sugar and Energy

The New Glucose Revolution Pocket Guide to Childhood Diabetes

The New Glucose Revolution Pocket Guide to Healthy Kids

■

The New Glucose Revolution Low GI Guide to Diabetes

The New Glucose Revolution Shoppers' Guide to GI Values 2006

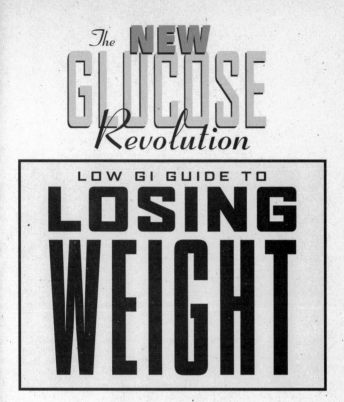

The NEW GLUCOSE *Revolution*

LOW GI GUIDE TO LOSING WEIGHT

Jennie Brand-Miller, Ph.D.
Stephen Colagiuri, M.D.
Kaye Foster-Powell, M. Nutr. & Diet.
with Johanna Burani, M.S., R.D., C.D.E.

Marlowe & Company
New York

THE NEW GLUCOSE REVOLUTION LOW GI GUIDE TO LOSING WEIGHT

Copyright © 2003 Jennie Brand-Miller, Stephen Colagiuri,
Kaye Foster-Powell, and Johanna Burani

Published by
Marlowe & Company
An Imprint of Avalon Publishing Group Incorporated
245 West 17th Street • 11th Floor
New York, NY 10011

This edition published in somewhat different form in Australia in 1998
under the title *Pocket Guide to the G.I. Factor and Losing Weight* by
Hodder Headline Australia Pty Limited. This edition published by
arrangement with Hodder Headline Australia Pty Limited.

The Library of Congress has cataloged the previous edition as follows:

The new glucose revolution pocket guide to losing weight / by Jennie
Brand-Miller ... [et al].
p. cm.
Rev. ed. of: The glucose revolution pocket guide to losing weight.
New York: Marlowe, 2000.
ISBN 1-56924-498-7
1. Reducing diets—Handbooks, manuals, etc. 2. Glycemic index—
Handbooks, manuals, etc. I. Title: Pocket guide to losing weight. II.
Brand Miller, Janette, 1952- III. Foster-Powell, Kaye. Glucose revolution
pocket guide to losing weight.
RM222.2.B66 2003
613.2'5—dc21   2003052732

This Edition
ISBN: 1-56924-336-0
ISBN-13: 978-1-56924-336-7

9 8 7 6 5 4 3

Designed by Pauline Neuwirth, Neuwirth & Associates, Inc.
Printed in Canada

CONTENTS

Introduction   ix

1 ▸ What This Book Can Do for You   1

2 ▸ Is Your Weight a Problem?   5

3 ▸ Why Are You Overweight?   9

4 ▸ Which Foods Affect Weight?   14

5 ▸ Understanding the Glycemic Index   21

6 ▸ How the Glycemic Index
    Can Help You Lose Weight   27

7 ▸ Exercise—We Can't Live without It   33

8 ▸ How Does Your Diet Rate?   39

9 ▸ Eating the Low-GI Way   47

10 ▸ Putting the Glycemic Index to Work
     in Your Day   52

11   The Low-GI Checklist   61
12   A Week of Low-GI Eating   69
13   GI Success Stories   79
14   Your Questions Answered   92
15   Cutting the Fat: Your A to Z Guide   96
16   Let's Talk Glycemic Load   103
17   A to Z GI Values   109
18   Low to High GI Values   127

     For More Information   145
     Glycemic Index Testing   147
     Acknowledgments   148
     About the Authors   149

INTRODUCTION

OBESITY IS NOW recognized as a serious health concern for a large majority of the American population. In the United States, nearly two-thirds of adults (64.5%) are overweight or obese. Even children are affected by unhealthy weight concerns: in 2000, approximately 15.3 percent of children (ages 6 to 11) and 15.5 percent of adolescents (ages 12 to 19) were overweight.

Our current obesity statistics result from *chronic* overconsumption of calorie-dense food portions (too many calories in), coupled with *chronic* inactivity (too few calories out). Our genes aren't changing; obesity results from an underactive lifestyle conducted within a food-toxic environment.

We need to tackle the problem on many fronts, including exercise and diet. The glycemic index (GI) can play an important role in weight management by helping to control appetite and insulin levels.

As we explain in *The New Glucose Revolution*, the glycemic index:

▶ is a scientifically proven measure of the effect carbohydrates have on blood-sugar (glucose) levels;
▶ helps you choose the right amount and right type
  of carbohydrate for your health and well being;
▶ provides an easy and effective way to eat a
  healthy diet and control fluctuations in blood
  glucose.

In this companion book to *The New Glucose Revolution*, we will show you how foods with low GI values can help you control your appetite, and help you choose the right foods for your lifestyle.

For more detailed information about the glycemic index and its many benefits, you should consult *The New Glucose Revolution*, or *The New Glucose Revolution Life Plan*, which provides even more recipes and practical information.

◀ 1 ▶

WHAT THIS BOOK
CAN DO FOR YOU

*W*HEN IT COMES to how to eat to lose weight, it is not simply a matter of reducing how much you eat. Research has shown that the type of food you feed your body determines what fuel it's going to burn for energy and what it's going to store as body fat. It has also revealed that certain foods are much more satisfying than others. Carbohydrates have the greatest effect on our blood-sugar levels, which determine at any given time how much energy we have, how mentally alert we are, *and* how hungry we feel. This is where the glycemic index (GI) comes into play. Low-GI foods have two very special advantages for people who want to lose weight:

▶ they fill you up and keep you satisfied for longer
▶ they help you burn more of your body fat and less of your body muscle

What Is the GI?

THE GLYCEMIC INDEX (GI) is a physiologically based measure of carbohydrate *quality*—a comparison of carbohydrates (gram for gram) based on their immediate effect on blood-glucose levels.

- Carbohydrates that break down quickly during digestion have high GI values. Their blood-glucose response is fast and high.
- Carbohydrates that break down slowly, releasing glucose gradually into the bloodstream, have a low GI.

For more information on the glycemic index, see page 25 or read *The New Glucose Revolution*.

If you are trying to lose weight, foods with low GI values will help you:

▶ increase your food intake without increasing your waistline
▶ control your appetite
▶ choose the right amount and the right kind of carbohydrate for your lifestyle

If you are overweight (or consider yourself overweight), chances are that you have looked at countless weight loss plans, books, and magazines offering a quick solution to losing weight. New diets pop up all the time. For the majority of people who are overweight, the "diets" don't work (if they did, there wouldn't be so many!).

At best—while you stick to it—a "diet" will reduce your calorie intake. At its worst, a "diet" will change your body composition, increasing its fat stores. This is because many diets promote reducing your carbohydrate intake to bring about quick weight loss. And you do lose weight—your body seems less "puffy" and your abdomen becomes less swollen, or even flat. But the weight you lose this way is mostly water (that was trapped or held in your muscles and liver, along with stored carbohydrate) and muscle (as it is broken down to produce glucose). Once you return to your former way of eating, your body has a little less muscle mass. With each desperate repetition of a diet you are more likely to lose more muscle. The change in body composition to less muscle and proportionately more fat makes weight control increasingly more difficult for you. So you see, there's nothing wrong with *you*, but there's *a lot wrong* with your dietary choices.

There's No Need to Feel Hungry When You Need to Lose Weight

WHEN YOU USE the GI as the basis for your food choices, there is:

- no need to overly restrict your food intake
- no need to obsessively count calories
- no need to starve yourself

■

This book is not another diet book!

■

This book offers you an everyday approach to weight management and shows you the scientific evidence demonstrating how you can best use the glycemic index to support your efforts at weight loss and permanent control.

- ▶ We show you how to put the GI into practice.
- ▶ We provide practical hints for changing your eating habits.
- ▶ We give you a week of low-GI, low-calorie menus plus a nutritional analysis for each menu and its GI values.
- ▶ We include an A to Z listing of more than four hundred foods with their GI values, carbohydrate, and fat content.

◀ 2 ▶

IS YOUR WEIGHT A PROBLEM?

CLARIFY IN YOUR own mind whether your weight really is a problem to you. Assess your current situation to understand exactly how you feel about your weight: what bothers you the most, and what are you willing to do about it?

Here are some questions you need to ask yourself:

- Do you think you are overweight?
- Do you think your weight is contributing to your poor health?
- Do you think your weight is impacting your daily life?
- Do you really want to lose weight?

ARE YOU OVERWEIGHT?

A commonly used weight-for-height chart called the Body Mass Index (BMI) indicates a range of weights considered healthiest for a particular height, but this reference isn't appropriate for everyone. Athletes, for example, may appear heavy in proportion to their height because of their muscle bulk, but this doesn't mean they are unhealthy. A large mass of body fat, on the other hand, *is* associated with health risk, especially when the fat is centrally located (waist, tummy, abdomen). Women often carry a lot of fat on their hips, thighs, and buttocks, giving them a pear shape. This fat carries little health risk. You can tell if you have too much fat on your middle by measuring your waist with a tape measure. A waist circumference bigger than 35 inches (females) or 40 inches (males) is too big.

■

Are you an apple or a pear?
Your waist circumference should be less than
35" (women) or less than 40" (men).

■

IS YOUR WEIGHT CONTRIBUTING
TO YOUR POOR HEALTH?

Centrally located fat is associated with a range of health problems. Among these are heart disease, diabetes, high blood pressure, gout, gallstones, sleep apnea (when breathing stops for a significant period of time; snoring is a good sign of this), and arthritis. Even if your fat is more uniformly distributed, it may still affect your health by limiting your physical mobility, creating strain and pain in your joints, and causing you to puff and pant with any physical exertion.

■

For the majority of people who are overweight, magazine "miracle diets" don't work. If they did, there wouldn't be so many of them.

■

IS YOUR WEIGHT HAVING AN IMPACT ON YOUR DAILY LIFE?

Aside from the physical side effects of being overweight, there are an equal number of emotional and psychological consequences. Your weight may inhibit you from meeting people, lower your self esteem, keep you from going swimming, make shopping for clothes a nightmare, stop you from playing with your children, prevent you from playing sports . . .

It is generally no fun being overweight.

IF YOU ARE currently eating healthy foods most of the time, with an occasional indulgence, and do physical activity for at least thirty minutes four to five times a week, then your present size and shape may be right for you.

DO YOU REALLY WANT TO LOSE WEIGHT?

The proportion of overweight people in our country is increasing, despite the expanding weight-loss industry and an ever-increasing range of diet foods. It is clear that the answer to weight management is not a simple one. Nor is losing weight easy to do. Using the glycemic index, however, can make it a little bit easier for you, because it tells you which foods satisfy hunger for a longer time, and which are the least likely to make you hungry and therefore, overeat. When you use the GI as the basis for your food choices, there is no need to:

- overly restrict your food intake
- obsessively count calories
- starve yourself

Learning which foods your body works best on is what using the GI is all about.

Taking control of aspects of your lifestyle that have an impact on your weight is worthwhile. You may not create a new body from your efforts, but you will feel better about the body you've got. Eating and exercising to feel your absolute best is the aim of the game.

3

WHY ARE YOU OVERWEIGHT?

For most of us, even without much conscious effort, our bodies maintain a constant weight, give or take a few pounds, even if it's higher than we'd like. We see this even despite huge variations in how much we sometimes eat. It's as if there's a weight our body wants to maintain. For many overweight people, this balancing of energy intake and output is operating at a higher threshold. So, regardless of all apparent efforts to control it—every fad diet, every exercise program, even some operations and medications—lost body weight is usually regained over the years.

Our weight is a result of how much we take in and how much we burn. So, if we take in too much and don't burn enough, we are likely to gain.

The question is: how much, of what, is too much?

The answer is not a simple one: not all foods are equal, and no two bodies are the same.

People are overweight for many different reasons. Research has made it clear that a combination of social, genetic, dietary, metabolic, psychological, and emotional factors combine to influence our weight.

In some people there is a genetic predisposition to weight gain. A child born to overweight parents is much more likely to be overweight than one whose parents were not overweight, for example. Studies in twins also provide evidence that our body weight and shape is at least partially determined by our genes.

Identical twins tend to be similar in body weight even if they are raised apart. Even twins adopted out as infants show the body-fat profile of their biological parents rather than that of their adoptive parents. These findings suggest that our genes are a stronger determinant of weight than our environment (which includes the food we eat).

It seems that information stored in our genes governs our tendency to store calories as either fat or as lean muscle tissue. Overfeeding a large group of identical twins confirmed that within each pair, weight gain was similar. However, the amount of weight gained between sets of identical twins varied greatly. From this, researchers concluded that our genes control the way our bodies respond to overeating. Some sets of twins gained a lot of weight, while others gained only a little, even though all were overconsuming an equivalent amount of excess calories.

All this isn't to say that if your parents are overweight, you should resign yourself to being overweight too. But it may help you understand why you have to watch your weight while other people seemingly don't have to watch theirs.

METABOLISM

Our genetic make-up also underlies our *metabolism* (basically, how many calories we burn per minute). Bodies, like cars, differ in this regard. A V-8 takes more fuel to run than a small four-cylinder car. A bigger body, generally, requires more calories than a smaller one. When a car is stationary, the engine idles—using just enough fuel to keep the motor running. When we are asleep, our engine keeps running (for example, our brain, heart, lungs, and so forth are still at work) and we use a minimum number of calories. This is our *resting metabolic rate*—the amount of calories we burn at rest. Most of it is necessary fuel for our large brains. When we start exercising, or even just moving around, the number of calories, or the amount of fuel we use, increases. The largest amount (around 70 pecent) of the calories used in a twenty-four-hour period, however, are those used to maintain our resting metabolic rate, because we spend most of our time at rest.

Measuring the Fuel We Need

CALORIES ARE A measure of the energy in food and the energy we require to keep us alive. Our bodies need a certain number of calories every day to keep our hearts beating and our brains working, just as a car needs so many gallons of gasoline to run for a day. Food and drink are our sources of calories. If we eat and drink too much, we store the additional calories as extra body fat and protein. If we consume fewer calories than we need, our bodies will break down fat and protein stores to make up for the shortfall.

Since our resting metabolic rate is how most of the calories we eat are used, it is a significant determinant of our body weight. The lower your resting metabolic rate, the greater your risk of gaining weight, and vice versa. We all know someone who appears to "eat like a horse" but is positively thin! We comment on their "fast metabolism," and we may not be far off the mark. Men's bodies are a good example, because they contain more muscle mass than women's and are calorically "expensive" to run; whatever body fat there is just goes along for the ride—it doesn't need calories to maintain it. Maintaining muscle mass by exercising is therefore important for weight control. New research also suggests that our genes dictate the fuel mix that we burn from minute to minute. A mix that contains *more energy derived from fat and less from carbohydrate* (even if the total energy burned per minute is the same) may aid in weight control.

IT'S NOT JUST GENETICS

Despite a genetic predisposition, you can only gain weight if you take in more energy than you use. We know that obesity has many causes—for example, eating too much, exercising too little, genetics, aging, and eating a high-fat diet and all play a part. But what it all boils down to is that if we take in too much (overeat) and don't burn up enough (don't exercise) we are likely to put on weight.

Factors Influencing Your Body Weight

CONSIDER WHICH OF the following factors may play a role for you:

- **Total food intake**
  Do you eat too many calories?

- **The balance of different nutrients**
  Do you eat a healthy, balanced diet?

- **Energy expenditure associated with movement**
  How much do you physically move in a normal day?

- **Energy expenditure associated with physical activity**
  How much planned activity do you do?

- **Resting metabolic rate**
  How much fuel does your body burn at rest?

- **Thermic response to food**
  How much fuel does your body waste as heat?

- **A body's preference to store excess calories as either fat or muscle**
  Do you have more fat or more muscle?

4

WHICH FOODS AFFECT WEIGHT?

So, IF YOU were born with a tendency to be overweight, why does it matter what you eat? The answer is that foods (or more correctly, nutrients) are not equal in their effect on body metabolism. In particular, the foods you eat dictate the fuel mix that you burn for several hours after eating. If you are burning more fat and less carbohydrate, even if the energy content of the food is the same, then chances are you'll be less hungry and less likely to gain body fat over the course of the day. Consequently, your choice of foods is critical for weight control.

Among all four major sources of calories in food (protein, fat, carbohydrate, and alcohol) fat has the highest energy density—more than twice that of carbohydrate and protein. A high-fat food contains a lot of calories in a relatively small amount of food; it is "energy-dense." A 3.5-ounce croissant made with wafer-thin layers of buttery pastry contains more than 400 calories. To eat the same amount of energy in the form of apples, you have to eat about three large apples. So, getting more energy—calories—than your body needs is relatively easy when you eat an energy-dense food.

Did You Know?

A FOOD'S "ENERGY DENSITY" (calories per gram) is more important to weight control than its fat content.

Some diets, such as traditional Mediterranean diets, contain quite a lot of fat (mainly from olive oil), but are still bulky, based as they are on large servings of fruit and vegetables, including foods such as beans.

Many new low-fat foods on the market are not bulky—they have the same number of calories as the original high-fat food. Examples include low-fat yogurt, ice cream, and sweet and salty snack products. So read the label—look for the energy content per cup or ounce or serving as your best guide to a food's "fattening" power.

You can eat quantity—just consider the quality!

During the 1990s, one of the most notable scientific findings was that high-fat foods were less satisfying than high-carbohydrate foods. For this reason, dieters were advised to eat fewer high-fat foods. The food industry responded to the call for more low-fat foods. Unfortunately, along the way, someone forgot to say that what really counts is the food's final caloric content. If a low-fat food has the same caloric density (calories per serving) as a high-fat food, then its calories are just as easy to overconsume. There are lots of low-fat products on the market that are no less calorically dense than the high-fat counterpart. The best examples are low-fat yogurt, ice cream, crackers, and cookies.

■

Think *energy density*, not high-fat or low-fat

■

Nutritionists have therefore had to fine-tune the message about diets for weight control:

- ▶ eating *bulky* food is more important than simply eating low fat
- ▶ the *type* of fat is more critical to long-term health
- ▶ the *type* of carbohydrate is as important as the amount

It was widely (and wrongly) believed for many years that sugar and starchy foods such as potato, rice, and pasta were the cause of obesity. Twenty years ago, every diet for weight loss advocated restriction of these carbohydrate-rich foods. One of the reasons for this carbohydrate restriction stemmed from the "instant results" of low-carbohydrate diets. If your diet is very low in carbohydrate, you will lose weight. The problem is that what you primarily lose is fluid, not fat. What's more, a low-carbohydrate diet depletes the glycogen stores—or reserved energy—in the muscles, thus making physical activity difficult and tiring.

Sugar has been blamed as a cause of obesity primarily because it is often found in high fat-foods, where it serves to make the fat more palatable and tempting.

Chocolate, which contains almost one-third of its weight in the form of fat, would be fairly unpalatable without the sugar.

On the whole, however, there is little evidence to condemn sugar or starchy foods, by themselves, as the cause of obesity. Overweight people show a preference for energy-dense foods rather than for foods high in sugar or starch. Their bodies have high energy requirements, even at rest, and the easiest way to satisfy their hunger is with high-energy foods. In a survey performed at the University of Michigan where obese men and women listed their favorite foods, men listed mainly fatty meats and women listed mainly cakes, cookies, and doughnuts. The unifying trait was a lot of energy-dense foods.

Counting the Calories

ALL FOODS CONTAIN calories. Often the calorie content of a food is considered a measure of how "fattening" it is. Of all the nutrients in food that we consume, carbohydrate and protein yield the fewest calories per gram.

carbohydrate	4 calories per gram
protein	4 calories per gram
alcohol	7 calories per gram
fat	9 calories per gram

Whether you are going to gain weight from eating a particular food really depends on how much that food adds to your total calorie intake in relation to how many calories you burn.

To lose weight, you need to eat fewer calories and burn more calories. If your total calorie balance does not change, there will be no change in your weight. People who consume a high-fat diet also tend to eat a high-calorie diet, because fatty foods yield more calories for the same weight of food than carbohydrate foods. This is why substituting low-fat foods for high-fat foods and focusing on reducing your total fat intake has the most potential to reduce your calorie intake and tip the energy balance in favor of weight loss.

Did You Know?

THE BODY LOVES to store fat. It is a way of protecting us in case of famine. But because we are in the midst of a calorie feast, we are building up our fat stores.

WHICH FOODS ARE MOST FATTENING?

Let's compare two everyday foods that are almost "pure" in the nutritional sense.

2 teaspoons of sugar   **vs.**   1 teaspoon of butter
(almost pure carbohydrate)   (almost pure fat)

They contain virtually the same number of calories.

32 calories   **vs.**   34 calories

This means that you can eat twice the volume of sugar as you can butter for the same number of calories! Look at these other examples:

- A small grilled T-bone steak (about the size of a slice of bread) has the same calories as three medium potatoes.
- Three slices of bread, thickly buttered, are equivalent to six slices of bread with no butter.
- Four Oreos have more calories than a 16 ounce-carton of 2% chocolate milk.
- Eating one piece of crumbed, fried chicken at lunch substitutes for the calories of six slices of bread (without butter).
- For every 1 cup of fried rice you eat, you could eat 2 cups of boiled rice.
- And if you're feeling extra hungry next time you stop for a coffee, consider that one glazed doughnut has the calories of three slices of lightly buttered raisin toast!

ARE YOU REALLY CHOOSING LOW-FAT?

There's a trick to food labels that it is worth being aware of when shopping for low-fat foods. These food-labeling specifications guidelines were enacted by the United States Department of Agriculture (USDA) in 1994:

Free: Contains a tiny or insignificant amount of fat, cholesterol, sodium, sugar, or calories; less than 0.5 grams (g) of fat per serving.

Low-fat: Contains no more than 3 g of fat per serving.

Reduced/Less/Fewer: These diet products must contain 25% less of a nutrient or calories than the regular product.

Light/Lite: These diet products contain one-third fewer calories than, or 50 percent the fat of, the original product.

Lean: Meats with "lean" on the label contain less than 10 g of fat, 4 g of saturated fat, and 95 milligrams (mg) of cholesterol per serving.

Extra lean: These meats have less than 5 g of fat, 2 g of saturated fat and 95 mg of cholesterol per serving.

In every case, the highest-fat foods have the highest calorie count. Because carbohydrate has about half the calories of fat, it is safer to eat more carbohydrate-rich food. What's more, your body is more likely to store fat and burn carbohydrate, so the calories contribute more to your "spread" when they come from fat.

■

No matter how excessive the amount of fat we eat, the body will always find space to store it.

■

◀ 5 ▶

UNDERSTANDING THE
GLYCEMIC INDEX

THE GI IS a scientifically validated tool in the dietary management of diabetes, weight reduction, and athletic performance.

Originally, research into the glycemic index of foods was inspired by the desire to identify the best foods for people with diabetes. But scientists are now discovering that the glycemic index has positive implications for everyone.

Eating to lose weight with low-GI foods is not difficult because you don't have to go hungry, and the weight loss you end up with is true fat release.

The real aim in losing weight is losing body fat and not going by what the scale says. Perhaps it would be better described as "releasing" body fat? After all, to lose something suggests that you hope to find it again someday!

∎

The GI is a ranking of foods based on their overall effect on blood-glucose levels

∎

UNDERSTANDING THE GI

The glycemic index concept was first developed in 1981 by Dr. David Jenkins, a professor of nutrition at the University of Toronto, Canada, to help determine which foods were best for people with diabetes. At that time, the diet for people with diabetes was based on a system of carbohydrate exchanges, which assumed that all carbohydrate foods produced the same effect on blood-glucose levels, even though earlier studies had already proven this was not correct. Jenkins was one of the first people to question this assumption and investigate how real foods behave in the bodies of real people.

Since then, scientists, including the authors of this book, have tested the effect of many foods on blood-glucose levels, and clinical studies in the United Kingdom, France, Italy, Australia, and Canada have all proven without doubt the value of the glycemic index.

The GI value of foods is simply a ranking of carbohydrates in foods according to their immediate impact on blood-glucose levels. Because carbohydrates have the greatest effect on blood-sugar levels, the glycemic index focuses on these foods. And why should you be concerned about blood-sugar levels? Because our blood-sugar level at any given time determines how much energy we have, how mentally clear we are, and how hungry we feel.

Today we know the GI values of hundreds of different food items that have been tested following the standardized method. We have included many of these values in the tables at the back of this book, but for more detailed information you should consult *The New Glucose Revolution* or *The New Glucose Revolution Shoppers' Guide to GI Values 2006*.

THE KEY IS THE RATE OF DIGESTION

Foods containing carbohydrates that break down quickly during digestion have the highest GI values. The blood-glucose response is fast and high (in other words, the glucose in the bloodstream increases rapidly). Conversely, foods that contain carbohydrates that break down slowly, releasing glucose gradually into the bloodstream, have low GI values.

For most people most of the time, the foods with low GI values have advantages over those with high GI values. This is especially true for those people trying to control their weight (or lose weight).

The higher the GI value of a food, the higher the blood-glucose levels after eating that food. Instant white rice (GI value 87) and baked potatoes (GI value 85) have very high GI values, meaning their effect on blood-glucose levels is almost as high as that of an equal amount of pure glucose (yes, you read it correctly).

Figure 1 shows the blood-glucose response to potatoes compared with pure glucose. Foods with a low GI value (such as lentils at 29) show a flatter blood-glucose response when eaten, as shown in Figure 2. The peak blood-glucose level is lower and the return to the more normal baseline levels is slower than with a high-GI food.

■

Low GI value = 55 or less
Intermediate GI value = 56 to 69
High GI value = 70 or more

■

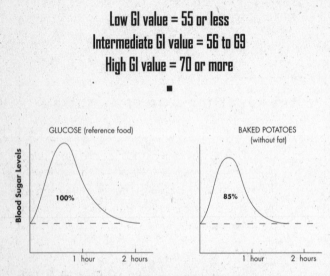

Figure 1. The effect of pure glucose (50 g) and baked potatoes without fat (50 g carbohydrate portion) on blood-glucose levels.

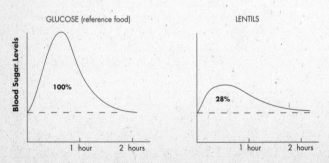

Figure 2. The effect of pure glucose (50 g) and lentils (50 g carbohydrate portion) on blood-glucose levels.

How We Measure the GI

PURE GLUCOSE PRODUCES the greatest rise in blood-glucose levels. Most foods have less effect when fed in equal carbohydrate quantities. The GI value of pure glucose is set at 100 and every other food is ranked on a scale from 0 to 100 according to its actual effect on blood-glucose levels.

1. An amount of food containing a standard amount of carbohydrate (usually 25 or 50 grams) is given to a volunteer to eat. For example, to test cooked spaghetti, the volunteer will be given 200 grams of spaghetti, which supplies 50 grams of carbohydrate (determined from food-composition tables).

2. Over the next two hours (or three hours if the volunteer has diabetes), we take a sample of their blood every 15 minutes during the first hour and thereafter every 30 minutes. The blood-glucose level of these blood samples is measured in the laboratory and recorded.

3. The blood-glucose level is plotted on a graph and the area under the curve is calculated using a computer program (Figure 3).

continued

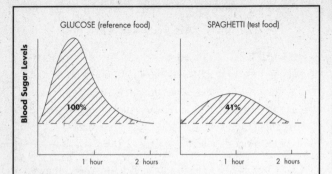

Figure 3. Measuring the GI value of a food
The test food and the reference food must contain the same
amount of carbohydrate. The usual dose is 50 grams, but
sometimes 25 grams is used when the portion size would be
otherwise too large. Even smaller doses such as 15 grams
have been used. The GI value is much the same whatever the
dose, because the GI number is simply a relative measure of
carbohydrate quality.

4. The volunteer's response to spaghetti (or whatever
   food is being tested) is compared with his or her
   blood-glucose response to 50 grams of pure glucose (the reference food).

5. The reference food is tested on two or three sep-
   arate occasions and an average value is calculated.
   This is done to reduce the effect of day-to-day
   variation in blood-glucose responses.

6. The average GI value found in eight to ten people
   is the GI value of that food.

6

HOW THE GLYCEMIC INDEX CAN HELP YOU LOSE WEIGHT

*O*NE OF THE toughest aspects of trying to lose weight can be feeling hungry all the time. But you don't have to have a gnawing, empty feeling when you're losing weight. Carbohydrates are natural appetite suppressants. Gram for gram of carbohydrate, those with a low GI value are the most filling and prevent hunger pangs for the longest amount of time.

In the past, it was believed that protein, fat, and carbohydrate foods, taken in equal quantities, satisfied our appetite equally. We now know from recent research that the satiating capacity—the degree to which foods make us feel full—of these nutrients is not equal.

Fatty foods, in particular, have only a weak effect on satisfying appetite relative to the number of calories they provide. This has been demonstrated clearly in experimental situations where people are asked to eat until their appetite is satisfied. They overconsume calories if the foods they are offered are high in fat. When high-carbohydrate and low-fat foods are offered, they consume fewer calories when given the opportunity to eat until satisfied. So, carbohydrate foods are the best for satisfying your appetite without oversatisfying your calorie requirement.

■

Low-GI foods fill you up and keep you satisfied for longer

■

In some research, people were given a range of individual foods that contained equal amounts of calories, and then their satiety responses were compared. We found that the most filling foods were those that contained fewer calories per gram, i.e. were the least energy-dense. This included potatoes, oatmeal, apples, oranges, and pasta. Eating more of these foods satisfies the appetite without providing excess calories. On the other hand, foods that provide a lot of calories per gram, like cookies, chocolate, and potato chips, were the least satisfying. These foods are more likely to leave us wanting more and to lead to what scientists call "passive overconsumption," i.e., overeating without realizing it.

After energy density, the second best predictor of satiety was a food's GI ranking—the lower the GI value, the more the food satisfied people's hunger. Indeed, there are now more than 17 studies that confirm low-GI foods are able to suppress hunger for longer than high-GI foods.

There are probably several mechanisms responsible for this.

- Low-GI foods remain longer in the small intestine, triggering receptors that tell the brain there's food still in the gut to be digested.
- High-GI foods may stimulate hunger because the rapid rise and then fall in blood-glucose levels appears to stimulate counterregulatory hormonal responses to reverse the decline.
- Stress hormones such as adrenalin and cortisol are released when glucose levels rebound after a high-GI food. Both hormones tend to stimulate appetite.
- Low-GI foods may be more satiating simply because they are often less energy-dense than their high-GI counterparts. The naturally high fiber content of many low-GI foods increases their bulk without increasing their energy content.

What's more, even when the calorie intake is the same, people eating low-GI foods may lose more weight than those eating high-GI foods. In one study, the investigators divided overweight volunteers into two groups: one group ate high-GI foods and the other, low-GI foods. The amount of calories, fat, protein, carbohydrate, and fiber in the diet was the same for both groups. Only the GI values of the diets were different. The low-GI group included foods like lentils, pasta, oatmeal, and corn in their diet and excluded high-GI foods like potato and white bread. After twelve weeks, the volunteers in the group eating low-GI foods had lost, on average, 20 pounds—4.5 pounds more than people in the group eating the diet of high-GI foods.

The most significant finding: the two diets affected blood levels of insulin completely differently. Low-GI foods resulted in lower levels of insulin circulating in

The Pancreas
Produces Insulin

THE PANCREAS IS a vital organ near the stomach, and its main job is to produce the hormone insulin. Carbohydrate stimulates the secretion of insulin more than any other component of food. The slow absorption of the carbohydrate in our food means that the pancreas doesn't have to work as hard and needs to produce less insulin. If the pancreas is overstimulated over a long period of time, it may become "exhausted," and Type 2 diabetes can develop in genetically susceptible people. Even without diabetes, high insulin levels are undesirable because they increase the risk of heart disease.

So this new, "more refined" way of eating brought with it higher blood-sugar levels after a meal and higher insulin responses as well. Our bodies need insulin for carbohydrate metabolism, but it has a profound effect on the development of many diseases. Medical experts now believe that high insulin levels are one of the key factors responsible for heart disease and hypertension. Insulin influences the way we metabolize foods, determining whether we burn fat or carbohydrate to meet our energy needs, and ultimately determining whether we store fat in our bodies.

Consequently, one of the most important ways in which our diet differs from that of our ancestors is the speed of carbohydrate digestion and the resulting effect on blood-sugar and insulin levels.

the bloodstream. Insulin is a hormone that is not only involved in regulating blood-sugar levels, it also plays a key part in when and how we store fat. High levels of insulin often exist in obese people, in those with high blood-fat levels (either cholesterol or triglyceride), and in those with heart disease. This study suggested that the low insulin responses associated with low-GI foods helped the body to burn more fat rather than store it.

■

**In looking at the diets of people
who want to lose weight,
the change required is often to
eat more.**

■

There are other reasons why low-GI diets might aid weight loss. When people first begin a diet, their metabolic rate drops in response to the reduction in food intake. One study, however, found that the metabolic rate had dropped less after one week on a low-GI diet than on a conventional high-carbohydrate diet. The same study suggested that the low-GI diet helped better to preserve lean body mass, which could explain the higher metabolic rate.

New findings also provide evidence that low-GI diets are able to reduce abdominal fat specifically. In a French study, overweight men were given in succession a high- and low-GI weight-maintaining diet (in random order), equivalent in energy and macronutrient composition. After five weeks on each diet, their body fat mass was measured using sophisticated X-ray methods. Those allocated to the low-GI diet had lost one pound of abdominal fat. There was no difference in subcutaneous fat (i.e., the fat under the skin). That evidence was backed up by a large observational study in Europe of people with Type 1 diabetes. It found that those who had naturally self-selected a low-GI diet had not only better blood-glucose control values, but the men in the group had lower waist circumferences, a good index of abdominal fat.

7

EXERCISE—
WE CAN'T LIVE WITHOUT IT

DIET ISN'T THE only way to manage diabetes. Because the disease stays with you for the rest of your life, taking good care of yourself requires adopting a few healthy lifestyle habits that must last a lifetime.

A multitude of changes in our living habits now mean that in both work and recreation we are more sedentary than ever. Our physical activity levels are now so low that we take in more calories than we burn off, causing us to gain weight. Luckily, exercise is our ticket back to healthy living.

Regular physical activity can reduce our blood-sugar levels, lower our risk of heart and blood-vessel disease, lower high blood pressure, increase stamina, reduce stress, and help us relax. It's a good idea for all of us.

■

To lose weight you need to eat fewer calories and burn more calories—and that means getting regular exercise and leading a more active lifestyle.

■

THE BENEFITS OF EXERCISE

Most people could tell you at least one health benefit of exercise (reduces blood pressure, lowers the risk of heart disease, improves circulation, and increases stamina, flexibility, and strength), but the most motivating aspect of exercise is feeling so good about yourself for doing it.

Exercise speeds up our metabolic rate. By increasing our caloric expenditure, exercise helps to balance our sometimes excessive caloric intake from food.

More movement makes our muscles better at using fat as a source of fuel. By improving the way insulin works, exercise increases the amount of fat we burn.

A low-GI diet has the same effect. Low-GI foods reduce the amount of insulin we need, which makes fat easier to burn and harder to store. Since it's body fat that you want to get rid of when you lose weight, exercise in combination with a low-GI diet makes a lot of sense!

HOW EXERCISE KEEPS BURNING CALORIES, EVEN WHEN YOU ARE AT REST

The effect of exercise doesn't stop when you do. People who exercise have higher metabolic rates, so their bodies

How to Get Moving

GETTING MORE EXERCISE doesn't necessarily mean daily aerobics classes and jogging around the block (although this is great if you want to do it). What it does mean is moving more in everyday living. It's the day-to-day things we do—shopping, ironing, chasing kids, walking from the train station—where we spend the bulk of our energy.

Since so much of our lifestyle is designed now to reduce our physical exertion, it's become very important to catch bursts of physical activity wherever we can, to increase our energy output. It may mean using the stairs instead of the elevator, taking a 10-minute walk at lunchtime, trotting on a treadmill while you watch the news or talk on the telephone, walking to the grocery store to get the Sunday paper, hiding the remote control, parking a half mile from work, or taking the dog for a walk each night. Whatever it means, do it. Even housework burns calories!

continue to burn more calories every minute, even when they're asleep!

Besides increasing your incidental activity, you will also benefit from some planned aerobic activity, which causes you to breathe more heavily and makes your heart beat faster. Walking, cycling, swimming, and stair climbing are just a few examples. You'll need to accumulate a total of at least 30 minutes of this type of activity five to six days a week.

Remember that reduction in body weight takes time. Even after you've made changes in your exercise habits, your weight may not be any different on the scale. (This is particularly true for women, whose bodies tend to adapt to increased caloric expenditure.)

Whatever it takes for you to burn more calories, do it. Try to regard movement as an opportunity to improve your physical well-being—not as an inconvenience.

USING THE GLYCEMIC INDEX WHEN YOU EXERCISE

We're talking about the everyday sort of moderate exercise that all of us should be doing. If you train physically hard a number of days a week and perhaps compete in sports, you should read *The Glucose Revolution Pocket Guide to Sports Nutrition*.

It is sometimes necessary with diabetes to eat extra carbohydrate when you exercise—depending on the type of diabetes you have and the type and amount of medication you take. Often, you won't want to increase your food intake—because the exercise is intended to burn off some earlier overconsumption! (For people with Type 1 diabetes, remember this will work only if you have enough insulin in your body and your blood sugars aren't too high to start with.)

You may need extra carbohydrate before you exercise, or, if the exercise is prolonged over an hour or more, you may need extra carbohydrate *while* you exercise, too. Whether or not you need to eat extra, and how much to eat depends on your blood-sugar level before, during, and after the exercise and how your body responds to the exercise—all of which you learn from experience.

8 Ways to Make Exercise Work for You

YOUR EXERCISE ROUTINE will bring you lots of benefits if you can:

1. appreciate its benefits
2. enjoy doing it
3. feel good about your ability to exercise
4. make it a normal part of your day
5. keep it inexpensive
6. make it accessible
7. stay safe while doing it
8. do it with someone

Discuss your situation and how best to manage it with a dietitian, diabetes educator, or doctor.

If you need to eat immediately before exercise to bring your blood sugar up during exercise, it makes sense to eat some high-GI carbohydrate, such as a slice of regular bread, a couple of cookies, or a ripe banana.

If you plan to eat your last meal or snack one to two hours before your exercise, it makes sense to eat a low-GI meal to sustain you through the exercise, such as a sandwich made with low-GI bread, low-fat protein such as turkey breast or boiled ham, a container of yogurt, or an apple.

If you need to eat something quickly after or during exercise to restore your blood-sugar level, use high-GI food—crispbread or rice cakes, a bowl of cornflakes or Rice Krispies, or a slice of watermelon, for example.

NOTE: Always remember to measure your blood sugar when you exercise to assess your body's response and judge your carbohydrate needs.

■

Exercise makes our muscles better at using fat as a source of fuel.

■

8

HOW DOES YOUR DIET RATE?

To MEET YOUR average daily nutrient requirements, you need to eat a certain amount of different types of foods. If you are trying to reduce your caloric intake, there is still a minimum amount of certain foods that you should be eating each day. These are:

BREADS/CEREALS/GRAIN FOODS— 6 SERVINGS OR MORE

1 serving means:
- 1 bowl breakfast cereal (1 ounce)
- ½ cup cooked pasta or rice
- ½ cup cooked grain such as barley or wheat
- 1 slice bread
- ½ roll or muffin

VEGETABLES—3 SERVINGS

1 serving means:
- 1 medium potato (about 5 ounces)
- ½ cup cooked vegetables such as broccoli or carrot (2 ounces)
- 1 cup raw leafy vegetables, such as lettuce

FRUIT—2-4 SERVINGS

1 serving means:
- 1 medium orange (7 ounces)
- 1 medium apple (5 ounces)
- ½ cup strawberries (4 ounces)

DAIRY FOODS—2 SERVINGS

1 serving means:
- 8 ounces low-fat milk
- 1½ ounces low-fat cheese
- 8 ounces low-fat yogurt

MEAT AND ALTERNATIVES—2 SERVINGS

1 serving means:
- 3 ounces cooked lean beef, veal, lamb, or pork
- 3 ounces lean chicken (cooked, excluding bone)
- 3 ounces fish (cooked, excluding bone)
- 2 eggs
- ½ cup cooked beans

If you prefer larger servings of meat, go ahead—just make sure it's lean. Protein is a very satiating nutrient.

HOW WELL ARE YOU EATING NOW?

Try keeping a detailed food diary for a week. Then, ooking at your diet record and using the serving-size guide below, estimate the number of servings of carbohydrate foods you had each day. For example, if you had a banana, two slices of bread and a medium potato, this counts as four servings of carbohydrate.

CARBOHYDRATE FOOD	ONE SERVING IS	HOW MANY DID YOU EAT?
Bread	1 slice	
Low GI:		
100% stoneground whole wheat, pumpernickel, sourdough, rye		
High GI:		
White, Italian, baguette		
Beverages	about ¾ cup (6 oz.)	
Low GI:		
Apple, tomato, grapefruit juice		
High GI:		
Cranberry juice cocktail, Gatorade		
Cooked breakfast cereals	½ cup cooked cereal	
Low GI:		
Old-fashioned oats, Apple and Cinnamon hot cereal (Con Agra)		
High GI:		
Instant Cream of Wheat, instant oatmeal		

CARBOHYDRATE FOOD	ONE SERVING IS	HOW MANY DID YOU EAT?
Fruit	a handful or 1 medium piece	
Low GI:		
Apples, bananas, oranges, grapes, peaches, strawberries		
High GI:		
Canned fruit cocktail, pineapple, watermelon		
Legumes	½ cup, cooked	
Low GI:		
Lentils, kidney, navy, pinto, lima beans		
Muffins, rolls	½ roll, muffin, or small bagel	
Low GI:		
Apple muffin, chocolate-butterscotch muffin		
High GI:		
English muffin, bagel, doughnut		
Noodles and rice	½ cup, cooked	
Low GI:		
Fettuccine, macaroni, tortellini		
High GI:		
Gnocchi, jasmine rice, arborio (risotto) rice		
Ready-to-eat breakfast cereals	1-ounce bowl	
Low GI:		
All Bran, Complete Bran Flakes		
High GI:		
Cheerios®, Grape-Nuts, Rice Krispies		
Starchy vegetables	½ cup, cooked or 1 cup, raw	
Low GI:		
Sweet potato, squash, peas		
High GI:		
Mashed potato, pumpkin, frozen french fries		
Total:		

Average the number of servings over all the days to come up with a daily average.

Low-GI Eating

LOW-GI EATING means making a move back to the high-carbohydrate foods that are staples in many parts of the world, especially whole grains (barley, oats, dried peas, and beans) in combination with breads, pasta, vegetables, fruits, and certain types of rice.

HOW DID YOUR SERVINGS RATE?

- Fewer than 4 servings a day: Poor.
- Between 4 and 8 servings a day: Fair, but you need to eat a lot more.
- Between 9 and 12 servings a day: Good, could need more if you are hungry.
- Between 13 and 16 servings a day: Great—this should meet the needs of most people.

HOW DID YOUR GI VALUES RATE?

- Fewer than 4 low-GI foods a day: Poor.
- Between 4 and 8 low-GI foods a day:
  Fair, but you need to eat a lot more low-GI foods.
- Between 9 and 12 low-GI foods a day:
  Good, but try to add more of these food choices.
- Between 13 and 16 low-GI foods a day:
  Great—you're eating a low-GI diet.

IS YOUR DIET TOO HIGH IN FAT?

Use this fat counter to tally up how much fat your diet contains. Do a tally for each day and then take an average. Using this fat counter, you will need to compare the serving size listed with your serving size and multiply the grams of fat up or down to match serving size. For example, if you estimate you might consume 2 cups of regular milk in a day, this supplies you with 16 grams of fat.

FOOD	FAT CONTENT (GRAMS)	HOW MUCH DID YOU EAT?
Dairy Foods		
Milk (8 oz.) 1 cup		
whole	8	
2%	5	
non-fat	0	
Yogurt (8 oz.)		
whole milk	7	
non-fat	0	
Ice cream, 2 scoops (1 cup)		
regular	15	
low-fat	3	
fat-free	0	
Cheese		
American, block cheese, 1 oz. slice	9	
reduced fat American cheese, 1 oz. slice	7	
low-fat slices (per slice)	3	
cottage, small curd, 2 tablespoons	3	
ricotta, whole milk, 2 tablespoons	2	
Cream, 1 tablespoon		
heavy	6	
light	5	
Sour cream, 1 tablespoon		
regular	3	
light	1	

FOOD	FAT CONTENT (GRAMS)	HOW MUCH DID YOU EAT?
Fats and Oils		
Butter, 1 teaspoon	4	
Oil, any type, 1 tablespoon (½ oz.)	14	
Cooking spray, per spray	0	
Mayonnaise, 1 tablespoon	11	
Salad dressing, 1 tablespoon	6	
Meat		
Beef		
steak, flank, lean only, 3½ oz.	10	
ground beef, extra-lean, 1 cup, 3½ oz., cooked, drained	16	
sausage, frankfurter, grilled, 2 oz.	16	
top sirloin, lean only, 3½ oz.	8	
Lamb		
rib chop, grilled, lean only, 3½ oz.	10	
leg, roasted, lean only, 3½ oz.	7	
loin chop, grilled, lean only, 3½ oz.	8	
Pork		
bacon, 3 strips, pan-fried	9	
ham, 1 slice, leg, lean, 3½ oz.	5	
steak, lean only, 3½ oz.	4	
leg, roasted, lean only, 3½ oz.	9	
loin chop, lean only, 3½ oz.	4	
Chicken		
breast, skinless, 3 oz.	4	
drumstick, skinless, 2 oz.	3	
thigh, skinless, 2 oz.	6	
½ barbecue chicken (including skin)	30	
Fish		
grilled fish, 1 average fillet, 4 oz.	1	
salmon, 3 oz.	3	
fish sticks, frozen, 4 baked	14	
fish fillets, 2, batter-dipped, frozen, oven-baked, 6 oz.		
regular	26	
light	10	

FOOD	FAT CONTENT (GRAMS)	HOW MUCH DID YOU EAT?
Snack Foods		
Chocolate bar, Hershey, 1½ oz.	13	
Potato chips, 1 oz. bag	10	
Corn chips, 1 oz. bag	10	
Peanuts, ½ cup (2½ oz.)	35	
French fries, 25 pieces	20	
Pizza, cheese, 2 slices, medium pizza	22	
Pie, apple, snack size	15	
Popcorn, fat and salt added, 3 cups	9	
Total:		

NOTE: The foods in this list have not been categorized as high or low GI since, with the exception of the snack foods, all other entries contain little or no carbohydrate, and thus are not ranked by the glycemic index.

How Did You Rate?

- **Less than 40 grams:** Excellent. 30 to 40 grams of fat per day is recommended for people trying to lose weight.
- **41 to 60 grams:** Good. A fat intake in this range is recommended for most adult men and women.
- **61 to 80 grams:** Acceptable if you are very active (doing hard physical work or athletic training). It is probably too much if you are trying to lose weight.
- **More than 80 grams:** You're probably eating too much fat, unless you're Superman or Superwoman!

9

EATING THE LOW-GI WAY

*L*OW-GI DIETS are easy to teach and easy to learn. The basic technique is to swap high-GI carbohydrates in your diet with low-GI foods. This could mean eating old-fashioned oatmeal at breakfast instead of cornflakes, whole-grain bread instead of white, or fruit in place of cookies, for example. Here are some key points that will help you put the glycemic index into practice. Remember:

▶ *The GI relates only to carbohydrate-rich foods*

The foods we eat contain three main nutrients—protein, carbohydrate, and fat. Some foods, such as meat, are high in protein, while bread is high in carbohydrate and butter is high in fat. It is necessary for us to consume a variety of foods (in varying proportions) to provide all three nutrients, but the glycemic index applies only to high-carbohydrate foods. It is impossible for us to measure a GI value for foods that contain negligible carbohydrate. These foods include meats, fish, chicken, eggs, cheese, nuts, oils, cream, butter, and most vegetables. There are other nutritional aspects that you could consider in choosing these foods; for example, the amount and type of fats they contain.

▶ *The glycemic index is not intended to be used in isolation*

The GI value of a food does not make it good or bad for us. High-GI foods such as a baked potato or white bread still make a valuable nutritional contribution to our diet. And low-GI foods such as pastry that are high in saturated fat are no better for us because of their low GI value. The nutritional benefits of different foods are many and varied, and it is advisable for you to base your food choices on the overall nutritional content of a food, particularly considering the saturated fat, salt, fiber, and GI values.

▶ *There is no need to eat only low-GI foods*

While most of us will benefit from eating carbohydrate with a low GI value at each meal, this doesn't mean consuming it to the exclusion of all other carbohydrate choices. When we eat a combination of low- and high-GI carbohydrate foods, such as hummus on toast, fruit and sandwiches, lentils and rice, potatoes and corn, the final GI value of the meal is intermediate. A high-GI food such as mashed potatoes is moderated by including a low-GI carbohydrate at the same meal, like adding kidney beans to a tossed salad, or a low-GI dessert such as yogurt.

Consider both the GI value of the food and the amount of carbohydrate it contains, i.e., the glycemic load

Because both the amount and type of carbohydrate are needed to predict blood-glucose responses to a meal, we needed a way to combine and describe the two. Researchers at Harvard University did this by coming up with the term "glycemic load." The glycemic load helps us predict what the effect of a particular carbohydrate food will be on our blood-glucose level after consuming that food. The glycemic load is greatest for those foods containing the most carbohydrate (like rice or spaghetti), especially when eaten in large quantities. The glycemic load is calculated simply by multiplying the GI value of a food by the amount of carbohydrate per serving and dividing by 100. We have included the glycemic load of foods in the tables at the back of this book.

■

A rule of thumb:
High-GI food + Low-GI food = Intermediate-GI meal

■

As with calories, the GI value is not precise. What GI values give you is a guide to lowering the GI values of the foods you eat throughout the day. A simple change can make a big difference. Look at the type of carbohydrate foods you eat and identify those you eat the most of (these have the greatest glycemic impact). Consider the high-carbohydrate foods you consume at each meal and replace at least one with a low-GI food (e.g., replace a white potato with a sweet potato). This will result in a significant reduction in the overall GI value of your diet. Look at the following table for substitution suggestions.

Low-GI Substitutes

High-GI Food	Low-GI Alternative
Bread, whole wheat or white	Whole-grain pumpernickel, sourdough, 100% stoneground whole wheat, whole wheat pita, sourdough rye
Processed breakfast cereal	Unrefined cereal such as rolled oats or or a low-GI processed cereal like All Bran™
Plain cookies and crackers	Cookies made with dried fruit and whole grains such as oats
Cakes and muffins	Make them with fruit, oats, whole grains
White potato	Substitute with new or sweet potatoes, or other starches such as corn, pasta, and legumes
Sticky or parboiled rice	Try Basmati or Uncle Ben's Converted rice, pearled barley, or noodles
Tropical fruits	Temperate-climate fruits such as bananas, apples, peaches, and nectarines

MAKING THE CHANGE

Some people change their diet easily, but for the majority of us, change of any kind is difficult. Changing our diet is seldom just a matter of giving up certain foods. A healthy diet contains a wide variety of foods, but we should try to eat them in appropriate proportions. If you are considering changes to your diet, keep these four guidelines in mind:

1. Aim to make changes gradually.
2. Attempt the easiest changes first.
3. Break big goals into a number of smaller, more easily achievable goals.
4. Accept lapses in your habits.

If you feel like you need some extra help, seek out some professional assistance from a dietitian.

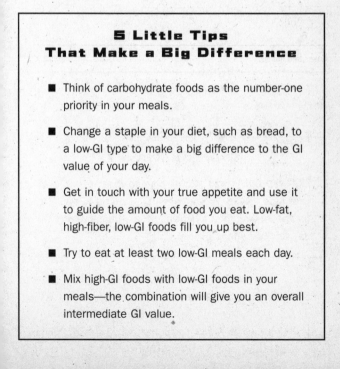

5 Little Tips
That Make a Big Difference

■ Think of carbohydrate foods as the number-one priority in your meals.

■ Change a staple in your diet, such as bread, to a low-GI type to make a big difference to the GI value of your day.

■ Get in touch with your true appetite and use it to guide the amount of food you eat. Low-fat, high-fiber, low-GI foods fill you up best.

■ Try to eat at least two low-GI meals each day.

■ Mix high-GI foods with low-GI foods in your meals—the combination will give you an overall intermediate GI value.

◀ 10 ▶

PUTTING THE GLYCEMIC INDEX
TO WORK IN YOUR DAY

ONCE YOU KNOW how to eat the low-GI way and which foods to reach for when you're hungry, it's easy to prepare low-fat, low-GI meals any time of the day. Here are a few ideas to get you started.

Did You Know?

SKIPPING BREAKFAST IS not a good way to cut back your food intake. Breakfast-skippers tend to make up for the missed food by eating more snacks during the day and more food overall.

BREAKFAST

▶ Try a cup of Kellogg's Complete® oat bran flakes with skim or 1% milk or yogurt.

▶ Eat a bowl of All-Bran™ or rolled oats (raw or cooked).

▶ If you prefer muesli or granola, keep it to a small bowl of a low-fat version—and check that it doesn't contain added fat.

▶ Have a slice of 100% stoneground whole-wheat bread or whole-grain pumpernickel (or 2 slices for a bigger person) with a tablespoon of jam or natural peanut butter or light cream cheese with sliced apple. Keep butter to a minimum, or use none at all.

▶ If you like a hot breakfast, try a boiled, scrambled, or poached egg with your toast.

---

7 Quick, Low-Fat, Low-GI Breakfast Ideas

1. Spread raisin toast with light cream cheese and top with sliced apple.

2. Toast stoneground whole-wheat bread and top with a slice of reduced-fat cheese.

3. Make old-fashioned oats with 1% milk; sprinkle with nuts and brown sugar.

4. Whip up a fruit smoothie with 1% milk, yogurt, a peach or a cup of frozen strawberries, and honey.

5. Top one 8-ounce container of light yogurt with grapes and raspberries.

6. Try a bowl of All-Bran™ with 1% milk and unsweetened canned pear slices.

7. Enjoy a sourdough English muffin with natural peanut butter and spreadable fruit.

Low-GI Lunches on the Go

1. Take some pita bread, spread it with hummus, and fill with tabouli.
2. Enjoy some chunky vegetable soup, thick with barley, beans, and noodles.
3. Cook a little pasta and mix with pesto, sun-dried tomatoes, or chopped fresh herbs and olive oil.
4. Put your favorite sandwich filling on dark rye bread (you can grill the sandwich if you like).
5. In a blender, whip up a fruit smoothie and couple it with a high-fiber apple muffin.
6. Mix fresh fruit with non-fat yogurt.
7. Have a cup of lentil soup with a sprinkle of grated cheese.
8. Steam or microwave a sweet potato and enjoy as is. Finish with some fruit and yogurt.
9. Couple a green salad with some bean salad, add whole-grain bread, and enjoy.

LUNCH

- Try a sandwich or roll with only a dab of butter. Choose 100% stoneground whole wheat, whole-grain pumpernickel, or any other bread made with lots of whole grains. Add plenty of sliced vegetables.
- For the filling, choose from boiled ham, lean roast beef, or chicken or turkey breast, or a slice of low-fat cheese, salmon, or tuna (in water), or an egg. An extra container of salad or vegetable soup will help to fill you up.

- Finish your lunch with a piece of fruit, fruit salad with low-fat yogurt, or low-fat chocolate or plain milk.

DINNER

- The basis of dinner should be carbohydrate foods. Take your pick from rice, pasta, sweet potato, couscous, bread, legumes—or a mixture.
- Then, add as many vegetables as you like, using a small amount of meat, chicken, or fish as a flavoring, rather than as the main ingredient.
- Use lean meat, such as London broil, veal, center-cut pork chop, trimmed lamb, chicken breast, fish fillets, or turkey. Red meat is a valuable source of iron—just choose lean types. A piece of meat, chicken, or fish that fits in the palm of your hand is your proper protein portion for dinner.
- If you prefer not to eat meat, a cup of cooked dried peas, beans, lentils, or chickpeas can provide protein and iron without any fat. At the same time they supply low-GI carbohydrate and fiber.
- Vegetarian products such as veggie burgers, tempeh, and tofu are based on high-protein legumes (such as soybeans and peanuts) and are good meat alternatives.
- Boost your fruit intake and get into the habit of finishing your meal with fruit—fresh, stewed, or baked. Or try a fruit ice, such as Dole Fruit Juice Bars.

7 Low-GI Dinner Ideas

1. Spaghetti with a lean meat sauce and large tossed salad, dressed with olive oil and vinegar.
2. Stir-fry chicken, meat, or fish with mixed green vegetables. Serve with Basmati rice or Chinese noodles.
3. Serve vegetable lasagna with salad.
4. Grill a steak and serve with a trio of low-GI vegetables—new potato, sweet corn, and peas.
5. Cook spinach and ricotta tortellini with garden vegetables and a tomato and mushroom sauce.
6. Wrap a fish fillet dressed with lemon, parsley, and garlic in foil. Bake and serve with mixed vegetables or salad.
7. Buy a barbecued chicken, steam sweet ears of corn, and toss a salad together.

DESSERTS: A LOW-GI FINISH

Although often overlooked, desserts can make a valuable contribution to your daily calcium and vitamin C intake when they are based on low-fat dairy foods and fruits. Recipes incorporating fruit for sweetness will have more fiber and lower GI values than recipes with sugar. What's more, desserts help signal to the brain the completion of eating, reducing the tendency for late-night nibbles.

If you don't have time to prepare a dessert, why not simply serve a bowl of fruit in season or have a baked apple? Remember, temperate-climate fruits such as apples, pears, peaches, plums, and nectarines tend to have lower GI values.

7 Quick and Easy Low-GI Desserts

1. Top low-fat ice cream with strawberries.
2. Stuff a whole apple with dried fruit and bake it.
3. Mix a fruit salad with low-fat yogurt.
4. Fruit crisp: Top cooked fruit with a crumbled mixture of toasted muesli, wheat flakes, a little melted butter, and honey.
5. Cook vanilla or chocolate pudding with skim or 1% milk and top with crushed walnuts or hazelnuts.
6. Fruited cream: Top canned fruit, such as peaches or pears, with low-fat ice cream, low-fat pudding, or sugar free Jell-O™.
7. Fruit strudel: Wrap chopped apple, raisins, currants, and spice in a sheet of filo pastry (brushed with milk, not fat) and bake as a strudel.

■

Low GI Value = 55 or less
Intermediate GI Value= 56 to 69
High GI Value = 70 or more

■

BETWEEN-MEAL SNACKS

It's normal to get hungry and want to snack between your usual "three squares." Luckily, when you eat the low-GI way, there's no prohibition on between-meal nibbles. It's a great way to eat the foods you love without gaining weight!

Just remember when you choose a between-meal bite to pick a low-fat snack with a low-GI value. For example, an apple with a GI value of 38 is better than a slice of white bread with a GI value of around 70, and will result in a smaller blood-sugar jump.

New evidence suggests that the people who graze, eating small amounts of food throughout the day at frequent intervals, may actually be doing themselves a favor. Spreading the food out over longer periods of time will flatten out the peaks and valleys of blood-glucose levels. So, snacking may be a good idea—as long as you don't overeat and gain weight.

Some snack foods with low GI values (such as peanuts, at 14) have a very high fat content and are not recommended for people trying to lose weight. As an occasional snack they are fine, especially because their fat is the healthier monounsaturated type. Just don't indulge in them every day. Remember, with peanuts, it's often hard to stop at just a handful!

SNACKING SUCCESS!

A recent study that compared people eating a diet of three meals a day with those who had three meals and three snacks showed that snacking stimulated the body to use up more energy for metabolism compared with concentrating the same amount of food into three meals. It's as if the more fuel you give your body, the more it will burn. Frequent small meals stimulate the metabolic rate.

5 Snacking Tips

1. It is important to include a couple of servings of dairy foods each day for your calcium needs. If you haven't had yogurt or cheese in any meals, you may choose to make a low-fat milkshake. One or two scoops of low-fat ice cream or pudding can also boost your daily calcium intake.

2. If you like whole-grain breads, an extra slice makes a very good choice for a snack. Other snacks can include toasted sourdough English muffin halves or a slice of raisin bread with a little butter.

3. Fruit is always a low-calorie option for snacks. You should try to consume at least three servings a day. It may be helpful to prepare fruit in advance to make it accessible and easy to eat.

4. Baked tortilla chips with lots of salsa is a low-calorie snack if you want something dry and crunchy.

5. Keep vegetables (such as celery and carrot sticks, baby tomatoes, florets of blanched cauliflower, or broccoli) ready prepared.

SUSTAINING SNACKS

- An apple
- An apple-and-oat-bran muffin
- A small bowl of cherries
- Ice cream (low-fat) in a cone
- Milk, milkshake, or smoothie (low-fat, of course)
- 2 or 3 small oatmeal cookies

- An orange
- Pita bread spread with apple butter
- One or 2 slices of raisin toast
- Whole-grain bread sandwich with your favorite filling
- A bowl of Raisin Bran™ with skim milk
- A handful of dried apricots
- Six to 8 ounces of light yogurt

10 Tips to Control Your Food Intake

1. Use hunger as your cue for eating—not the time of day.
2. Eat a low-GI carbohydrate food when you are hungry—these foods are the most satiating.
3. Slow down when you eat to give your stomach a chance to give the signal to your brain that it is full.
4. When you are thinking about eating, ask yourself how hungry you really are. Delay eating for 30 minutes—true hunger will return.
5. Don't buy foods that you don't want to eat.
6. Indulge in the occasional treat. Lollipops or hard candies are more filling than chocolates.
7. Give yourself time to make changes in your habits. It takes about six weeks for your taste buds to readjust.
8. Once you have served your meal or snack, put the remaining food away, so it is out of sight.
9. Keep busy during the day.
10. Don't restrain your food intake excessively—use the eating checklists in Chapter 8 (pages 39–46) to make sure you eat enough.

THE LOW-GI CHECKLIST

*G*OING GROCERY SHOPPING? Bring this list with you. It will help you choose low- and intermediate-GI foods quickly and easily.

BREADS

100% stoneground whole-wheat
100% Whole Grain, Natural Ovens
Flatbread, Indian
Happiness, Natural Ovens
Hearty 7 Grain
Hunger Filler, Natural Ovens
Muesli, made from mix
Natural Wheat, Natural Ovens
Pita, whole-wheat
Pumpernickel, whole-grain
Rye
Sourdough

Sourdough rye
Soy & Linseed, machine mix
Spelt, multigrain

BREAKFAST CEREALS

All-Bran with Extra Fiber™
Bran Buds with Psyllium™
Bran Buds™, Kellogg's
Bran Chex™, Kellogg's
Bran flakes™, Complete®, Kellogg's
Cereal, hot, apple and cinnamon, ConAgra
Cream of Wheat™, regular, Nabisco
Frosted Flakes™, Kellogg's
Fruit Loops, Kellogg's
Just Right™, Kellogg's
Life™, Quaker Oats
Muesli, natural
Muesli, toasted
Nutrigrain™, Kellogg's
Oat bran
Oat bran, raw
Oatmeal, old-fashioned, cooked
Puffed Wheat, Quaker Oatss
Raisin Bran™, Kellogg's
Rice bran
Special K™, Kellogg's

COOKIES AND CAKES

Biscuits, Social Tea™
Bread, banana
Cake, chocolate, with chocolate frosting

Cake, pound
Cake, sponge
Cake, vanilla
Cookies, Arrowroot
Cookies, Hearty Oatmeal, FIFTY50
Cookies, oatmeal
Cookies, Oatmeal, Sugar Free, FIFTY50
Cookies, shortbread
Muffin, apple cinnamon, from mix*
Wafers, vanilla, creme filled, FIFTY50

DAIRY PRODUCTS AND ALTERNATIVES

Custard, homemade
Ice cream, regular
Milk, low-fat, chocolate, with aspartame
Milk, low-fat, chocolate, with sugar
Milk, skim
Milk, whole
Mousse, butterscotch, low-fat, Nestlé
Mousse, chocolate, low-fat, Nestlé
Mousse, French vanilla, low-fat, Nestlé
Mousse, hazelnut, low-fat, Nestlé
Mousse, mango, low-fat, Nestlé
Mousse, mixed berry, low-fat, Nestlé
Mousse, strawberry, low-fat, Nestlé
Pudding, instant, chocolate, made with milk
Pudding, instant, vanilla, made with milk
Soy milk, reduced-fat
Soy milk, whole
Yogurt, low-fat, fruit, with aspartame

*Foods containing fat in excess of American Heart Association guidelines. Use these only once in a while and in small amounts.

Yogurt, low-fat, fruit, with sugar
Yogurt, non-fat, French vanilla, with sugar
Yogurt, non-fat, strawberry, with sugar

FRUIT AND FRUIT PRODUCTS

Apple, fresh
Apricot, fresh
Banana, fresh
Cantaloupe, fresh
Cherries, fresh
Figs, dried
Fruit cocktail, canned
Grapefruit, fresh
Grapes, fresh
Kiwi, fresh
Mango, fresh
Orange, fresh
Papaya, fresh
Peach, canned in natural juice
Peach, fresh
Pear, canned in pear juice
Pineapple, fresh
Pear, fresh
Plum, fresh
Prunes, pitted
Raisins/sultanas
Strawberries, fresh
Strawberry jam

GRAINS

Barley, cracked
Barley, pearled

Barley, rolled
Buckwheat
Buckwheat groats
Bulgur
Corn, canned, no salt added
Corn, fresh
Couscous
Rice, arborio (risotto)
Rice, Basmati
Rice, brown
Rice, Cajun Style, Uncle Ben's®
Rice, Garden Style, Uncle Ben's®
Rice, Long Grain and Wild, Uncle Ben's®
Rice, parboiled, Converted, white, cooked 20–30 min,
     Uncle Ben's®
Rice, parboiled, Long Grain, cooked 10 minutes,
     Uncle Ben's®

JUICES

Apple, with sugar or artificial sweetener
Carrot, fresh
Grapefruit, unsweetened
Pineapple, unsweetened
Tomato, canned, no added sugar

LEGUMES

Beans, baked, canned
Beans, butter, dried and cooked
Beans, kidney, canned
Beans, lima, baby, frozen
Beans, mung, cooked

Beans, navy, dried and cooked
Beans, pinto, cooked
Beans, soy, canned
Chickpeas/garbanzo beans, canned
Lentils, green, dried and cooked
Lentils, red, dried and cooked
Peas, black-eyed
Peas, split, yellow, cooked

Note: Canned legumes have higher GI values than the boiled varieties because the temperatures and pressures used in the canning process increase the digestibility of the starch. But, canned legumes are still an excellent low-fat, high-fiber, nutrient-rich low-GI choice!

NOODLES AND PASTA

Capellini
Fettuccine, egg
Gluten-free noodles, cornstarch
Instant noodles
Linguine, thick, fresh, durum wheat, white, fresh
Linguine, thin, fresh, durum wheat
Macaroni, plain, cooked
Mung bean, Lungkow beanthread
Ravioli
Rice, dried, cooked
Rice, fresh, cooked
Spaghetti, cooked 5 minutes
Spaghetti, cooked 10 minutes, Barilla
Spaghetti, cooked 22 minutes
Spaghetti, protein-enriched, cooked 7 minutes
Spaghetti, whole wheat

Spirali, cooked, durum wheat
Star pastina, cooked 5 minutes
Tortellini
Udon, plain, reheated 5 minutes
Vermicelli

SNACK FOODS

Apple Cinnamon snack bar, ConAgra
Cashews
Chocolate bar, milk, Cadbury's
Chocolate bar, milk, Dove®, Mars
Chocolate bar, milk, Nestlé
Chocolate bar, white, Milky Bar®
Chocolate bar, Snickers®
Corn chips, plain, salted, Doritos™
M&M's®, peanut
Nougat
Nutella®, chocolate hazelnut spread
Peanut Butter & chocolate-chip snack bar
Peanuts
Pecans
Potato chips, plain, salted
Twix® Cookie Bar, caramel

SOUPS

Black bean, canned
Green pea, canned
Lentil, canned
Minestrone, canned, ready-to-serve
Tomato, canned

STARCHY VEGETABLES

Corn
Peas
Potato, new, canned
Potato, sweet
Yam

VEGETABLES

Artichokes
Avocado
Beet
Bok choy
Broccoli
Cabbage
Carrots, peeled, cooked
Cassava (yucca), cooked with salt
Cauliflower
Celery
Corn, canned, no salt added
Corn, sweet, cooked
Cucumber
French beans (runner beans)
Leafy greens
Lettuce
Peas, frozen cooked
Pepper
Potato, boiled/canned
Potato, new, canned
Squash
Taro
Yam

◀ 12 ▶

A WEEK OF LOW-GI EATING

*H*ERE'S A WHOLE week of healthy, low-calorie menus with all the benefits of low-GI foods. Each menu is designed to be:

- **low in fat.** Eating less fat is an easy way to reduce your energy intake. To lose weight, aim for a daily fat intake of 30 to 50 grams. Skim or 1% milk and minimal added fat are used throughout the menus.
- **high in carbohydrate with a low GI Value.** Carbohydrates, especially those with low GI values, are the most satisfying for your appetite. It's also the best fuel for your body; at least half the calories each day come from carbohydrate. This means eating around 200 grams a day at a minimum.

- ▶ **low in calories.** You'll lose weight if you reduce your calorie intake, but it's important not to go too low. The daily average of these menus is approximately 1,300 to 1,500 calories.
- ▶ **nutritionally balanced.** Including a large variety of foods, but in the right proportions, makes you more likely to meet your nutrient needs.

These menus are not a prescription! Use them for ideas and as a guide to amounts and types of foods for a low-calorie diet.

MARGARINE: FRIEND OR FOE?

You'll notice that in some of the meals below, we suggest using light margarine. As you may know, many margarines are sources of trans fats, which can raise cholesterol levels and have been implicated in increased risk of heart attacks and possibly even breast cancer. Luckily, not all margarine is created equal! Some products now on store shelves clearly boast that they are trans-fat free (look for those). Here are some other guidelines Johanna Burani, M.S., R.D., C.D.E., suggests you follow to avoid these unhealthy fats:

- ▶ Buy margarine by the tub, not the stick
- ▶ Look for "light," "low-fat," "non-fat," or "fat-free" on the label
- ▶ Make sure the first ingredient says "liquid," such as "liquid corn oil" or "liquid safflower oil"

Try tub margarines that contain plant sterol esters.

Note: We understand that the portions listed in these menus may seem small—at least at first. But the good news is, as long as you're moving *toward* eating smaller portions (and we're showing you the appropriate portion sizes for the calories), you'll be making progress. The proof of that progress will show up in your weight and in your blood sugar, cholesterol, and blood pressure numbers.

MONDAY

GI:	49
Total Energy:	1474 cal.
Fat:	34 g
Carbohydrate:	232 g
Fiber:	32 g

■

Breakfast: Oatmeal and fruit

Cook or microwave a bowl of oatmeal using ½ cup old-fashioned oats, with 8 ounces skim milk. Add ½ cup natural applesauce. Sprinkle with cinnamon and 1 tablespoon sugar.

Alternative: Soften the oats for a little while in cold 1% milk and eat them as muesli, topped with a sliced banana.

Morning snack: Eight dried apricot halves and a cup of lemon tea or coffee

Lunch: Ham and salad sandwich

Make a ham sandwich with 2 slices of 100% stone-ground whole-wheat bread, 2 ounces boiled ham, lettuce, tomato, mustard, grated carrot, and sprouts. Finish with a small juicy apple.

Afternoon snack: Two oatmeal cookies

Dinner: Vegetable lasagna and salad

See *The New Glucose Revolution* for our low-fat, low-GI recipe for Vegetable Lasagna (p. 126). Serve with a side salad of your choice. For dessert, try a fresh fruit salad and a ½-cup scoop of low-fat ice cream.

Evening snack: Fun-size Snickers (or other) chocolate bar

TUESDAY

GI:	47
Total Energy:	1543 cal.
Fat:	47 g
Carbohydrate:	202 g
Fiber:	31 g

■

Breakfast: Peanut butter toast
  Spread a slice of 100% stoneground whole-wheat toast with 1 tablespoon natural peanut butter. Finish off with a pear or other fresh fruit.

Morning snack: A small bunch of grapes

Lunch: Soup and bread
  Have a 1-cup bowl of split pea and ham soup with 3 stoneground wheat thins. Complete the meal with an orange.

Afternoon snack: Enjoy a hot or iced latte, made with 8 ounces 1% milk

Dinner: Spaghetti with lean meat sauce
  Serve ⅓ cup sauce over 1 cup cooked spaghetti. Accompany with a large tossed salad.

Evening snack: A small handful of peanuts (1 ounce). If you think you might have trouble sticking to this amount, make sure you buy peanuts in the shell—at least that will slow you down!

WEDNESDAY

GI:	53
Total Energy:	1267 cal.
Fat:	19 g
Carbohydrate:	202 g
Fiber:	32g

■

Breakfast: Cereal and fruit

Two-thirds of a cup of All Bran with extra fiber™, topped with 6 ounces 1% milk. Add 4 slices of unsweetened canned pears or accompany with a 4-ounce glass of apple juice.

Morning snack: Handful (about 10) of sourdough pretzel nuggets

Lunch: Pasta and sauce

Toss a cup of boiled pasta with about ⅓ cup of bottled tomato and mushroom sauce. Add a tossed green salad drizzled with fat-free dressing.

Afternoon snack: Small scoop (½ cup) non-fat ice cream in a cup or cone

Dinner: Tuna casserole with rice

Make a quick tuna casserole using a 3-ounce can of tuna, onion, celery, and peas combined in a cheese sauce. Serve with 1 cup Basmati or long-grain rice, seasoned with fresh parsley.

Evening snack: A cup of fresh fruit salad

THURSDAY

GI:	48
Total Energy:	1394 cal.
Fat:	38 g
Carbohydrate:	90 g
Fiber:	23 g

■

Breakfast: Muesli and yogurt
  Pour 2 ounces non-fat milk over ½ cup natural muesli. Top with 4 ounces light fruit yogurt and 4 ounces fresh or unsweetened canned peaches.

Morning snack: Two oatmeal cookies and a cup of tea or coffee

Lunch: Grilled cheese sandwich
  Make a grilled cheese and tomato sandwich on toasted 100% stoneground whole-wheat bread. Finish with a crunchy green apple.

Afternoon snack: Toast a slice of raisin bread and spread lightly with ½ tablespoon light margarine. Drink a cup of light, no-sugar-added hot chocolate with it.

Dinner: Pork and vegetables
  Grill or broil a 3-ounce center loin pork cutlet, basting with a favorite marinade if desired. Serve with 3 steamed new potatoes, a small ear of corn on the cob, ½ cup broccoli and ½ cup green beans.

Dessert: Have ½ cup sliced strawberries and 1 scoop of low-fat ice cream and finish the meal with a cup of flavored decaf coffee.

FRIDAY

GI:	44
Total Energy:	1385 cal.
Fat:	29 g
Carbohydrate:	203 g
Fiber:	27 g

■

Breakfast: Tea and toast
One half grapefruit with a teaspoon of sugar, followed by 2 slices of pumpernickel bread toast spread with 1 tablespoon light cream cheese and 1 ounce salmon. Finish with a cup of tea.

Morning snack: A cup of sugar-free hot chocolate

Lunch: Tuna-stuffed pita pocket
Cut a 2-ounce whole wheat pita in half, fill each half with shredded lettuce and diced fresh tomatoes. Top each half with 2 heaping tablespoons of low-fat tuna salad.

Afternoon snack: An 8-ounce container of light yogurt

Alternative: Fruit smoothie
Blend together a nectarine (or other seasonal fruit) with 4 ounces of light yogurt.

Dinner: Beef stroganoff with mushrooms and wine
Small serving of casserole (containing approximately 3 ounces cubed tenderloin). Serve with 1 cup of boiled fettucine, ½ cup of green beans, and baby carrots.

Evening snack: Small bag (1 ounce) of potato chips

SATURDAY

GI:	45
Total Energy:	1511 cal.
Fat:	31 g
Carbohydrate:	216 g
Fiber:	23 g

■

Breakfast: Egg and bagel

A hard- or soft-boiled egg and a sourdough English muffin spread with 1 tablespoon light margarine. Finish with an 8-ounce cup of non-fat, no-sugar-added hot chocolate.

Morning snack: Low-fat honey 'n' oats granola bar

Lunch: Vegetable grain toss

Mix 1 cup of a cooked commercial whole-grain mix (such as Lipton Rice and Sauce with Cajun Style Beans, Casbah Wheat Pilaf or Near East Barley Pilaf) with 1 cup of fresh or frozen cooked vegetables. Toss.

Afternoon snack: A small low-fat ice cream cone.

Dinner: Lemon flounder with vegetables

Broil or poach 2 5-ounce flounder fillets in lemon juice and white wine. Season with herbs and spices as desired. Serve with a cup of boiled Basmati or Uncle Ben's Converted™ Rice, ½ cup of steamed broccoli and ½ cup of carrots.

Evening snack: A large pear, poached in white wine and cardamom

SUNDAY

GI:	52
Total Energy:	1294 cal.
Fat:	34 g
Carbohydrate:	180 g
Fiber:	24 g

■

Breakfast: Sunday smoothie

Blend ¾ cup of 1% milk, ¼ cup plain non-fat yogurt, ½ teaspoon honey, ½ cup frozen berries and a dash of nutmeg in a blender for a delicious, nourishing drink.

Morning snack: A thin slice of homemade nut bread with tea or coffee

Lunch: Pita pizza

Toast 2-ounce whole-wheat pita. Cover top with tomato sauce, basil, oregano, and 2 ounces part-skim shredded mozzarella. Bake or grill until the cheese melts. Add in a large tossed salad topped with your favorite fat-free dressing. Finish up with an apple, orange, or a handful of grapes.

Afternoon snack: Handful of baked tortilla chips and salsa

Dinner: Steak and salad

Cook a 4-ounce sirloin steak to your liking. Have it with 3 boiled new potatoes, ½ cup of white bean salad (may use a canned mixed bean salad). Add a green salad, dressed with 1 tablespoon vinaigrette.

Evening snack: A generous wedge of honeydew (about 2 cups)

◀ 13 ▶

GI SUCCESS STORIES

*J*UST IN CASE you're not yet convinced that a low-GI diet can help you lose weight, dietitian Johanna Burani, M.S., R.D., C.D.E., offers these three real-life examples from her own practice. Many of Johanna's patients have lost weight, controlled their diabetes and gained overall better health by choosing a low-GI way of life.

CASE STUDY #1
"Marge"

Age:	33
Height:	5'4¾"
Weight:	246 pounds

(clinically defined as "morbidly obese")

Background:

Marge is a single mother who smokes one pack of cig-arettes a day, drinks alcoholic beverages socially, and does no deliberate exercise.

Marge's "before" diet:

Breakfast: Fried bacon and eggs, 2 slices white toast with butter, water

Lunch (which she skips once or twice a week): usually eats at a fast-food restaurant. Typical meal: Quarter-pounder with cheese, large French fries, diet Coke

Late-afternoon snack: Handful of chocolate kisses, 5 or 6 Ritz crackers, Cheddar cheese

Dinner: Steak, baked potato with butter, small por-tion of broccoli, instant pudding

Late-night snack: Large bowl of ice cream

Marge's "Before" Nutritional Analysis:

Calories:	3600
Carbohydrate:	185 g (21%)
Protein:	157 g (18%)
Fat:	246 g (61%)
GI:	74

Johanna's nutritional assessment:

To lose weight, Marge had to decrease her caloric intake, and specifically the amount of fat she was eating. To improve the nutrient balance of her meals and snacks, she would need to include at least five servings of fruits and vegetables, and two or three servings of dairy foods each day.

GI-specific counseling:

It was Marge's high fat intake that kept her feeling full. Grossly decreasing her dietary fat would leave her hungry, since her carbohydrate choices had high GI values.

By increasing her carbohydrate calories and selecting low-GI foods, Marge could achieve the same sense of prolonged satiety (feelings of fullness) that fat provides, with less than half the calories!

Marge's new, low-GI menu:

Breakfast: Two slices 100% stoneground whole-wheat toast, 2 tablespoons natural peanut butter, 8 oz. 1% milk and a handful of grapes

Snack: Six to 8 oz. of light yogurt (plain or fruit flavored)

Lunch: Two-ounce pita, 2 oz. roasted turkey breast, lettuce, and tomato, large mixed salad with fat-free dressing, an orange, and decaf diet beverage

Dinner: Shrimp teriyaki stir fry: ⅔ cup Uncle Ben's Converted™ Rice, 4 oz. shrimp, at least 1 cup Oriental vegetables (fresh or frozen), 3 oz. cherries and herbal diet iced tea or water

Snack: Eight oz. 1% milk and a large oatmeal cookie

Marge's "After" Nutritional Analysis:	
Calories:	1600
Carbohydrate:	231 g (56%)
Protein:	93 g (23%)
Fat:	38 g (21%)
GI:	43

Marge's winning results:

Marge has been following her low-GI meal plan for two and a half years. So far, she has lost 72 pounds (current weight: 174 pounds). Her goal weight is 160 pounds.

Marge's comments:

"I can't believe I'm never hungry. This is such an easy way to lose weight—and I don't consider this a diet. I love how I look and feel!"

CASE STUDY #2
"Annie"

Age:	7
Height:	3'8"
Weight:	80 pounds

(clinically defined as "morbidly obese")

Background:

Annie is a second grader who lives at home with her parents and a younger sibling. No one else in her family has a weight problem. Annie's pediatrician advised Annie's mother to seek nutritional guidance from an R.D. to help her gradually lose approximately 10 pounds over the next year. Annie's mother admitted to a lack of nutritional knowledge, but emphasized the whole family's willingness to implement Johanna's recommended dietary changes.

Annie's "before" diet:

Breakfast: A ¾ oz. serving of Rice Chex™ and 4 oz. 1% milk

Snack: An 8 oz. glass of milk and a breakfast bar

Lunch: Turkey breast on a small roll, ½ cup instant
  mashed potatoes with gravy and 8 oz. 1% milk
Snack: Two Oreo cookies and an ice cream sandwich
Dinner: Small bowl of commercial chicken noodle
  soup with 5 saltines and a cup of orange soda
Late-night snack: One-half orange

Annie's "Before" Nutritional Analysis:	
Calories:	1700
Carbohydrate:	251 g (60%)
Protein:	64 g (15%)
Fat:	46 g (25%)
GI:	70

Johanna's nutritional assessment:
  Annie's diet contains multiple nutritional problems.

- Her morbid obesity at such a young age predis-
  poses her to weight-related health problems later
  in life if she doesn't make changes now.
- While her milk consumption appears to meet at
  least the minimal calcium needs of a seven-year-
  old child, her other quality protein foods (meat,
  fish, eggs, and so on) may be lacking on some days.
- Her fiber intake is inadequate because she eats
  very little fruit, vegetables, and whole grains; her
  consumption of vitamins and minerals is also likely
  to be inadequate.
- She complains of being too tired to play after
  school.
- She is hungry all the time.

GI-specific counseling:

By decreasing her excessive carbohydrate intake (most of which are high-GI foods), and substituting low-GI fruits, vegetables, and whole grains, Annie will start consuming fewer—yet still enough—calories, have more energy, and feel fuller, longer. And in the process, Annie will enjoy a balanced meal plan to meet the demanding nutrient needs of a growing seven-year-old!

Annie's new, low-GI menu:

Breakfast: Three-quarters cup Quaker Life™ cereal, 4 oz. 1% milk and ½ banana

Snack: One-half sandwich bag of green grapes (about 17), 4 oz. 1% milk

Lunch: A ham-and-Swiss sandwich on 2 slices rye bread with lettuce, tomato, and mustard, 10 baby carrots, 4 oz. 1% milk

Snack: Four Social Tea™ biscuits, 4 oz. 1% milk

Dinner: Chicken leg, breaded without the skin, ½ cup mashed sweet potato, ½ cup green beans vinaigrette, ½ cup natural applesauce, 4 oz. 1% milk

Snack: One-half cup low-fat pudding

Annie's "After" Nutritional Analysis:

Calories:	1400
Carbohydrate:	196 g (58%)
Protein:	74 g (22%)
Fat:	31 g (20%)
GI:	51

Annie's winning results:

Over the past eight months, Annie has lost seven pounds and has grown an inch. Her weight is finally back on the height/weight growth chart again. Annie's doctor wants her to continue her current dietary regimen and check back in six months.

Annie's mother's comments:

Annie's mother is thrilled to see her little girl less moody and more energetic. She is particularly happy that meal and snack times are no longer tumultuous battles.

CASE STUDY #3
"Bill"

Age:	43
Height:	5'10"
Weight:	245 pounds

(clinically defined as "morbidly obese")

Background:

Bill works as a stockbroker and commutes three hours to and from his office each day. For exercise, he bikes or walks for 30 to 45 minutes, three or four times a week. He doesn't drink much water and drinks alcohol on the weekends. Over the past two years, Bill has gained 35 pounds. Bill's diet revealed a huge disparity between what he eats on "good" and "bad" days: Below is one of Bill's "bad" days.

Bill's "before" diet:

Breakfast: Two slices of rye toast with jelly, 2 cups of coffee

Snack: A large cheese Danish and a cup of coffee

Lunch: A bowl of chicken soup, roast beef and provolone hoagie, cole slaw, large order of French fries, large cup of low-fat frozen yogurt with M&Ms™ topping and 2 large glasses of sweetened iced tea

Dinner: Broiled chicken breast stuffed with spinach, large portion of eggplant parmesan, ½ large French baguette, and wine

Late-night snack: Ten peanut butter Girl Scout cookies with 16 oz. of skim milk

---

Bill's "Before" Nutritional Analysis:

Calories:	5500
Carbohydrate:	544 g (40%)
Protein:	244 g (18%)
Fat:	258 g (42%)
GI:	73

Johanna's nutritional assessment:

The only chance Bill has to lose weight is to reduce his calorie intake to a reasonable level and to eat a consistent number of calories from day to day. By varying his food consumption so drastically (from 1,300 calories on "good" days to more than 5,000 on "bad" days), he was actually programming his body to store more fat!

GI-specific counseling:

Because his days are long, Bill needs nutrient-dense, sustaining meals and snacks. Replacing nearly 75 percent of his excessive fat calories with low-GI foods would give him the satiety he was accustomed to for a small fraction of the calories.

Bill's new, low-GI menu:

Breakfast: One and ⅓ cups Fiber One cereal, 8 oz. of skim milk and 1 whole grapefruit

Lunch: A roast beef sandwich with lettuce and tomato in a large pita, large tossed salad with fat-free dressing, 8 oz. skim milk

Snack: A 1½ cup portion of fresh fruit salad

Dinner: One cup steamed brown rice, 4 oz. pork tenderloin (roasted), 1 cup spinach with garlic and olive oil, tossed salad (if desired), water or small glass of wine, 4 oz. natural applesauce

Snack: Three graham crackers, 8 oz. skim milk

Bill's "After" Nutritional Analysis:

Calories:	2000
Carbohydrate:	251 g (50%)
Protein:	112 g (22%)
Fat:	62 g (28%)
GI:	47

Bill's winning results:

In nine months, Bill lost 45 pounds, bringing him to his goal weight of 200 pounds. Four years later, he is happily maintaining his goal weight!

Bill's comments:

"I like the foods I'm eating. The best part, though, is that I'm not so draggy when I get home at night. I still have energy to enjoy my family."

CASE STUDY #4
"Ruth"

Age:	42
Height:	5'
Weight:	212 pounds
	(severely obese)

Background:

Ruth is a soon-to-be-married woman who works as a bookkeeper. Other than an annoying reflux problem, gall bladder surgery six years ago, and a metal plate in her right ankle after a nasty fall in her home, Ruth enjoys good health. She does complain, though, of always being tired. This is why she decided it was time to tackle her weight problem. The first big step she took was to sign up at an all-women's gym and commit to a 30-minute workout four times a week. Next she was ready to attack her diet.

Ruth's "before" diet:

Breakfast: Two hard-boiled eggs, 4-6 oz. cottage cheese, ¼ cup cashews, water

Lunch: 6 oz. grilled chicken breast, green salad with low-fat dressing, water

Dinner: Can of organic vegetable soup, 4 oz. low-fat cheese, 2 slices whole-wheat bread, water

Ruth's "Before" Nutritional Analysis:

Calories:	1400
Carbohydrate:	65 g (18%)
Protein:	112 g (32%)
Fat:	79 g (50%)
GI:	56

Johanna's nutritional assessment:

Ruth's average caloric intake does not appear to be the cause of her current weight problem. She is certainly not overeating. But 50 percent of the calories in her diet come from fat! Such a high-fat diet has never promoted permanent weight loss for anyone, and it wasn't doing it for Ruth, either. While she does choose healthier high-protein foods, she's not getting adequate carb calories, which would supply her with energy and, if the carbs are chosen correctly, sustain that energy level while quieting her appetite. She needs a well-balanced, high-fiber diet structured around whole-grain, unrefined staple foods, fruits, vegetables, and low-fat dairy products.

GI-specific counseling:

To start balancing her daily calories, Ruth can include a fruit serving with each meal, milk or yogurt at breakfast and as a snack before going to the gym. She should also incorporate low-GI breads, pasta, rice, and sweet potatoes to provide energy calories to her body throughout the day. These changes will squeeze out the space for so many fat calories, providing a healthier nutrient and energy balance.

Ruth's new, low-GI menu:

Breakfast: One-half cup old-fashioned rolled oats cooked in 8 oz. plain low-fat soy milk, 4 oz. natural applesauce, water

Snack: Four Social Tea biscuits

Lunch: Two slices 100% stoneground whole-wheat bread, 2 tablespoons soy nut butter, 1 cup steamed cauliflower, ¾ cup berries, water

Dinner: Soy burger on 100% whole-wheat bun, 2 cups string beans with margarine added

Snack: An apple

Ruth's "After" Nutritional Analysis:

Calories:	1500
Carbohydrate:	204 g (54%)
Protein:	84 g (22%)
Fat:	40 g (24%)
GI:	43

Ruth's winning results:

Ruth has lost 23 pounds in the past year without ever relapsing into a weight gain or old eating habits. She's also lost her reflux problem. She's at the gym at least five times a week now (although she admits it's a struggle to find the time while planning her wedding). When she takes those vows, Ruth will be wearing a wedding dress two sizes smaller than just a year ago.

Ruth's comments:

"I wasn't looking for another diet. I knew I wanted a lifestyle change. Filling my day with well-balanced-high-carb, low-GI meals has ended my search. I'm very happy."

14

YOUR QUESTIONS ANSWERED

Why are diets that disregard widely accepted nutritional guidelines so fashionable right now?

Several best-selling books have been published promoting high-protein diets and generating a lot of publicity. They have been seized upon as a viable weight-loss panacea. But the fact is: diets that limit major food groups do not work over the long haul.

What are the side effects of a high-protein diet?

The body cannot process large quantities of protein, so excess waste is produced that can overburden the kidneys. Not only can some high-protein diets make existing kidney problems worse, but they also can cause mild renal failure to progress faster. Some high-protein diets are also harmful for elderly people and anyone with high blood pressure or diabetes. High-protein, high-fat diets can lead to high cholesterol and heart disease, and can increase the risk of heart attack. Further, some high-protein diets reduce the intake of important vitamins, minerals, fiber, and trace elements. They also lack fiber, which may lead to constipation.

Why do people on high-protein diets shed pounds?

Because the diets make people lose water weight. Overweight people need to lose body fat—not muscle or water. And the way to do this is by eating a balanced diet of low-GI carbohydrates and burning more calories than we take in.

How do high-carbohydrate, low-GI diets help people to lose weight?

- Because low-GI diets lower insulin levels, over the long term you'll burn more—and store less—fat. (Insulin determines how much fat we store and burn.)
- You're less likely to overeat low-GI carbohydrates, because they're bulky and filling. Consider them natural appetite suppressants!
- A low-GI diet offers you plenty of food choices, so you're less likely to feel deprived. Unlike diets that restrict certain foods, a low-GI diet is easy to live with.

Can I still lose weight eating as much carbohydrate as I want?

Possibly not. We recommend a high carbohydrate intake and a low fat intake. While carbohydrate is not usually stored as fat, if you are eating more total energy than your body requires, then the carbohydrate will be used as a source of fuel in preference to fat. This would have the effect of limiting the breakdown of body fat stores. The idea is to eat enough energy in total to satisfy your appetite (using low-GI foods helps) and nutritional requirements, but not more than you need. An increase in your activity level will help burn up body fat as it is used as an additional fuel.

I've always heard that sugar is fattening. Is it?

No. Sugar has no special fattening properties—in fact, it is no more likely to be turned into fat than any other carbohydrate. Sugar, which you'll often find in foods high in calories and fat, may sometimes seem to be "turned into fat," but it's the total number of calories you're consuming rather than the sugar in those calorie-dense foods that may contribute to new stores of fat.

What effect does fiber have on the GI value?

There is no simple answer to this question. Dietary fiber is not one chemical constituent, as fat and protein are. It is composed of many different sorts of molecules. Fiber can lower the GI value in some foods and not in others, depending on its physical form.

Soluble fiber tends to be viscous (thick and jelly-like) and can slow down digestion. Thus, the presence of soluble fiber in such foods as oats and legumes may contribute to their low GI values. Purified psyllium added to foods slows down digestion because it is also viscous.

Insoluble fiber in flours is finely ground and often doesn't slow digestion. Whole-wheat bread and white bread have similar GI values. Brown pasta and brown rice have values similar to their white counterparts.

Sometimes insoluble fiber acts as a physical barrier that prevents the enzymes from attacking the starch. Whole (intact) grains of wheat, rye, and barley have lower GI values than cracked grains.

◀ 15 ▶

CUTTING THE FAT:
YOUR A TO Z GUIDE

*A*S WE HAVE said constantly throughout this book, it is important to eat a high-carbohydrate and low fat diet. The following practical tips that we have set out in an easy A to Z format will help you reduce the fat content of some of your favorite recipes while lowering their GI value.

Alcohol
Although excessive alcohol consumption can be fattening, as an ingredient in a recipe, alcohol itself won't create a high-calorie dish. Alcohol evaporates during cooking, so you lose the calories and are left with the flavor. A little wine in a sauce can give a delicious flavor, and sherry in an Asian-style marinade is essential.

Bacon
Bacon is a valuable ingredient in many dishes because of the flavor it offers. You can make a little bacon go a long

way by trimming off all fat and chopping it finely. Lean ham is often a more economical and leaner way to go. In casseroles and soups, a ham bone imparts a fine flavor without much fat.

Cheese

Several commonly used cheeses, such as American, Cheddar, and blue, contain more than 70 percent of their calories as fat. Although there are a number of fat-reduced cheeses available, many of these lose a lot in flavor for a small reduction in fat. It is worth comparing fat per ounce between brands to find the tastiest one with the lowest fat content. Alternatively, a sprinkle of a, very tasty grated cheese or Parmesan may do the job.

Part-skim ricotta and cottage cheeses are lower-fat alternatives to butter on a sandwich. It's worth trying some fresh part-skim ricotta from a deli—you may find the texture and flavor more acceptable than that of the ricotta available in containers in the supermarket. Flavored cottage cheeses are ideal low-fat toppings for crackers. Try ricotta in lasagna instead of a creamy white sauce.

Cream and sour cream

Keep to very small amounts, as these are high in saturated fat. Substitute non-fat sour cream, which tastes very similar to the full-fat variety. A 16-ounce container of heavy cream can be poured into ice-cube trays and frozen, providing small servings of cream easily when you need it. Adding one ice-cube block (1 oz.) of cream to a dish adds only 5½ grams of fat.

Dried beans, peas, and lentils

These are all low in fat and very nutritious. Incorporating them in a recipe, perhaps as a partial substitution for meat, will lower the fat content of the finished product. Canned beans, chickpeas, and lentils are now widely available. They are very convenient to use and a great time saver. They are comparable in food value to the dried ones that you soak and cook yourself.

Eggs

Be conscious of eggs in a recipe, as they can add fat. Sometimes just the beaten egg white can be substituted for the whole egg, or use real egg substitute.

Filo pastry

Unlike most other pastry, filo (also known as phyllo) is low in fat. To keep it that way, brush between the sheets with skim milk instead of melted butter when you prepare it. Look for it in the freezer section of the supermarket with other prepared pastry and use it as a strudel wrap.

Grilling

Grill or broil, rather than fry, tender cuts of meat, chicken and fish. Marinating first will add flavor, moisture, and tenderness. Grilling vegetables is a great way to bring out their flavor to the utmost.

Health food stores

Health food stores can be traps for the unwary. Check out the high-fat ingredients, such as hydrogenated vegetable oil, nuts, coconut, and palm kernel oil in products such as granola bars, fruit bars, and "healthy" cakes (even if made with whole-wheat flour) that they stock on their shelves.

Ice cream
A source of carbohydrate, calcium, riboflavin, retinol, and protein. Low-fat varieties have lower glycemic index values. Definitely a nutritious and icy treat.

Jam
A tablespoon of jam on toast contains far fewer calories than a pat of butter. So, enjoy your jam and give fat the flick!

Keep jars of minced garlic, chili, or ginger in the refrigerator to spice up your cooking in an instant.

Lemon juice
Try a fresh squeeze with ground black pepper on vegetables instead of a pat of butter. Lemon juice provides acidity that slows gastric emptying and lowers the GI value.

Milk
Many people dislike skim milk, particularly when they taste it on its own or in their coffee. However, you can use skim milk in a recipe and no one will notice—and the fat savings is great. For convenience you might want to keep powdered skim milk in the pantry, which can be made up to the desired quantity when you need it. It will taste more like fresh milk if you mix the powder and water according to directions and refrigerate the milk overnight before using it. Ultrapasteurized (or shelf stable) milk is handy in the cupboard, too.

Nuts

Nuts are valuable for their vitamin E content, but they are also high in fat. To keep the fat content of a recipe low, the quantity of nuts has to be small.

Oil

Most of our recipes call for no more than two teaspoons of oil. Any polyunsaturated or monounsaturated oil is suitable. Cooking spray or brushing oil lightly over the base of the pan is ideal. If you find the amount of oil insufficient, cover your pan, or add a few drops of water and use steam to cook the ingredients without burning. It is a good idea to invest in a nonstick frying pan if you don't have one.

Pasta

A food to eat more of and a great source of carbohydrate and B vitamins. Fresh or dried, the preparation is easy. Just boil in water until tender or "al dente," drain, and top with a dollop of pesto, tomato sauce, or a sprinkle of Parmesan and pepper. There are many wonderful pasta cookbooks now available, and it's definitely worth investing in one to find all sorts of exciting ways to prepare this fabulous low-GI food. Pasta may appear in your menu as a side dish to meat, as noodles in soup, as a meal in itself with vegetables or sauce, or even as an ingredient in a dessert.

Questions

Ask your dietitian for more recipe ideas. (See page 145 in "For More Information" for guidance on finding a dietitian near you.)

Reduce the fat content of ground beef by browning it in a nonstick pan, then placing the meat in a colander and pouring boiling water through it to wash away the fat. Return to the pan to continue cooking. It is a good idea to buy the better-quality ground beef with less fat.

Stock

If you are prepared to go to the effort of making your own stock—good for you! Prepare it in advance, refrigerate it, then skim off the accumulated fat from the top. Prepared stock is available in long-life cartons and cans in the supermarket. Stock cubes are another alternative. Look for brands that have reduced salt.

To sauté

Heat the pan first, brush with the recommended amount of oil (or less), add the food and cook, stirring lightly over a gentle heat.

Underlying the need for fat is a need for taste. Be creative with other flavorings.

Vinegar

A vinaigrette dressing (1 tablespoon vinegar and 2 tablespoons of oil) with your salad can lower the blood-sugar response to the whole meal by up to 30 percent. The best types of vinegars for this purpose are red and white wine vinegar. You can also use lemon juice.

Weighing

What's the weight of the meat you're buying? Start noticing the weight that appears on the butcher's scales or package label and consider how many servings it will give you. With a food such as steak, which is basically all edible meat, 4 to 5 ounces per serving is sufficient. One pound is more than enough for four portions. Choose lean cuts of meat and trim away the fat before cooking or before you put it away. Alternate meat or chicken with fish once or twice a week.

Yogurt

Yogurt is a valuable food in many ways. It is a good source of calcium, "friendly bacteria," protein, and riboflavin, and, unlike milk, is suitable for people who are lactose-intolerant. Low-fat plain yogurt is a suitable substitute for sour cream. If you're using yogurt in a hot sauce or casserole, add it at the last minute and do not let it boil, or it will curdle. It is best if you can bring the yogurt to room temperature before adding it to the hot dish. To do this, mix a small amount of yogurt with a little sauce from the dish, then stir this mixture back into the bulk of the sauce.

Zero fat

Eating zero fat is unhealthy, so speak with a dietitian about how to get just the right amount you need. Our bodies need essential fatty acids that can't be synthesized and must be supplied in the diet. Fat does add flavor—use it to your advantage.

◀ 16 ▶

LET'S TALK GLYCEMIC LOAD

*I*N ADDITION TO the GI values we provide in this book, our tables also include the glycemic load (GL) value for average-sized food portions. Taken together, the glycemic index and glycemic load provide you with all the information you need to choose a diet brimming with health-boosting foods.

GLYCEMIC LOAD 101

A food's glycemic load results from the GI value and carbohydrate per serving of food. When we eat a carbohydrate-containing meal, our blood glucose first rises, then falls. The extent to which it rises and remains high is critically important to our health and depends on two things: the *amount* of a carbohydrate in the meal and the *nature* (GI value) of that carbohydrate. Both factors equally determine blood-glucose changes.

Researchers at Harvard University came up with a way of combining and describing these two factors with the term "glycemic load," which not only provides a measure of the level of glucose in the blood, but also the insulin demand produced by a normal serving of the food. Researchers measure GI values for fixed portions of foods containing a certain amount of carbohydrate (usually 50 grams). Then, as people eat different-sized portions of the same foods, we can work out the extent to which a certain portion of food will raise the blood-glucose level by calculating a glycemic load value for that amount of food.

To calculate glycemic load, multiply a food's GI value by the amount of carbohydrate in a particular serving size, then divide by 100.

■

Glycemic load = (GI Value x carbohydrate per serving) ÷ 100

■

For example, a small apple has a GI value of 40 and contains 15 grams of carbohydrate. Its glycemic load is $(40 \times 15) \div 100 = 6$. A small 5-ounce potato has a GI value of 90 and 15 grams of carbohydrate. It has a glycemic load of $(90 \times 15) \div 100 = 14$. This means one small potato will raise your blood-glucose level higher than one apple.

■

Low GL = 10 or less
Intermediate GL = 11–19
High GL = 20 or more

■

How GI Values Affect Glycemic Load

THE GLYCEMIC LOAD is greatest for those foods that provide the highest-GI carbohydrate, particularly those we tend to eat in large quantities. Compare the glycemic load of the following foods to see how the serving size, as well as the GI value, help to determine the glycemic response:

Rice, 1 cup	Spaghetti, 1 cup
Carbohydrates: 43	Carbohydrates: 40
GI: 83	GI: 44
GL: 36	GL: 18
$(83 \times 43) \div 100 = 36$	$(44 \times 40) \div 100 = 18$

Some nutritionists argue that the glycemic load is an improvement on the glycemic index because it provides an estimate of both quantity *and* quality of carbohydrate (the GI value gives us just quality) in a diet. In large Harvard studies, however, researchers were able to predict disease risk from people's overall diet, as well as its glycemic load. Using the glycemic load strengthened the relationship, suggesting that the more frequently we consume high-carbohydrate, high-GI foods, the worse it is for our health. Carbohydrate by itself has no effect—in other words, there was no benefit of low-carbohydrate intake over high-carbohydrate intake, or vice versa.

Remember that the GL values we provide are for the standardized (nominal) portion sizes listed. If you eat a different portion size, then you'll need to calculate another GI value. Here's how: First, determine the size of your portion, then work out the available carbohydrate content of this weight (this value is listed next to the GL), then multiply by the food's GI value. For example, the nominal serving size listed for bran flakes is ½ cup, the available carbohydrate is 18 grams, and the GI value is 74. So the GL for ½-cup serving of bran flakes is (74 × 18) ÷ 100 = 13. If, however, you normally eat 1 cup of bran flakes, you'd need to double the available carbohydrate (18 × 2 = 36), and the GL for your larger cereal portion would be (74 × 36) ÷ 100 = 27. These numbers show that the larger portion of cereal releases a larger quantity of glucose into the bloodstream.

We urge you not to make the mistake of using the glycemic load alone. If you do, you might find yourself eating a diet with very little carbohydrate but a lot of fat—especially saturated fat—and excessive amounts of protein. For your overall health, the fat, fiber, and micronutrient content of your diet is also important. A dietitian can guide you further with healthy food choices.

THE TABLES

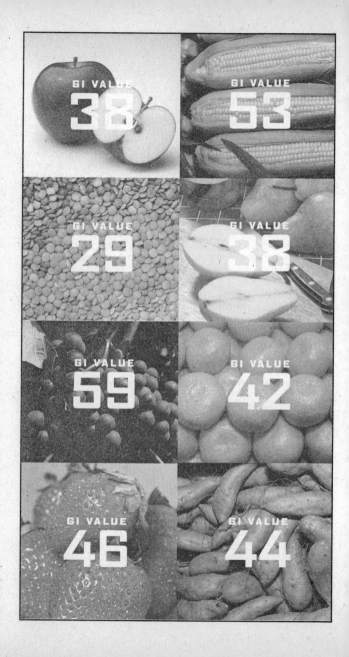

◀ 17 ▶

A TO Z
GI VALUES

*T*HE TABLE IN this section will help you find a food's glycemic index value quickly and easily, because we've listed the foods alphabetically.

The list provides not only the food's GI value but also its glycemic load (GL = (carbohydrate content × GI value) ÷ 100). We calculate the glycemic load using a "nominal" serving size as well as the carbohydrate content of that serving—both of which we've also listed. That way, you can choose foods with either a low GI value or a low glycemic load. If your favorite food is both high-GI and high-GL, you can either cut down the serving size or dilute the GL by combining it with very-low-GI foods, such as rice and lentils.

For the first time, we've also included foods that have very little carbohydrate; their GI value is zero, indicated by [0]. Many vegetables, such as avocados and broccoli, and protein foods such as chicken, cheese, and tuna, fall into the low- or no-carbohydrate category. Most alcoholic beverages are also low in carbohydrate.

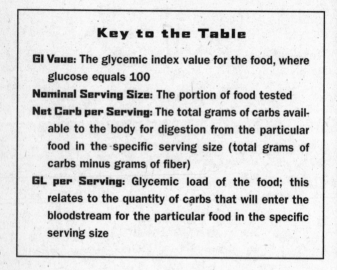

Key to the Table

GI Value: The glycemic index value for the food, where glucose equals 100

Nominal Serving Size: The portion of food tested

Net Carb per Serving: The total grams of carbs available to the body for digestion from the particular food in the specific serving size (total grams of carbs minus grams of fiber)

GL per Serving: Glycemic load of the food; this relates to the quantity of carbs that will enter the bloodstream for the particular food in the specific serving size

FOOD	GI Value	Nominal Serving Size	Net Carb per Serving	GL per Serving
A				
All-Bran®, breakfast cereal	30	½ cup	15	4
Almonds	[0]	1.75 oz	0	0
Angel food cake, 1 slice	67	1/12 cake	29	19
Apple, dried	29	9 rings	34	10
Apple, fresh, medium	38	4 oz	15	6
Apple juice, pure, unsweetened, reconstituted	40	8 oz	29	12
Apple muffin, small	44	3.5 oz	41	18
Apricots, canned in light syrup	64	4 halves	19	12
Apricots, dried	30	17 halves	27	8
Apricots, fresh, 3 medium	57	4 oz	9	5
Arborio, risotto rice, cooked	69	¾ cup	53	36
Artichokes (Jerusalem)	[0]	½ cup	0	0
Avocado	[0]	¼	0	0
B				
Bagel, white	72	½	35	25
Baked beans	38	⅔ cup	31	12
Baked beans, canned in tomato sauce	48	⅔ cup	15	7
Banana cake, 1 slice	47	⅛ cake	38	18
Banana, fresh, medium	52	4 oz	24	12
Barley, pearled, cooked	25	1 cup	42	11
Basmati rice, white, cooked	58	1 cup	38	22
Beef	[0]	4 oz	0	0
Beer	[0]	8 oz	10	0
Beets, canned	64	½ cup	7	5
Bengal gram dahl, chickpea	11	5 oz	36	4
Black bean soup	64	1 cup	27	17
Black beans, cooked	30	⅘ cup	23	7
Black-eyed peas, canned	42	⅔ cup	17	7

[0] indicates that the food has so little carbohydrate that the GI value cannot be tested. The GL, therefore, is 0.

FOOD	GI Value	Nominal Serving Size	Net Carb per Serving	GL per Serving
Blueberry muffin, small	59	3.5 oz	47	28
Bok choy, raw	[0]	1 cup	0	0
Bran Flakes™, breakfast cereal	74	½ cup	18	13
Bran muffin, small	60	3.5 oz	41	25
Brandy	[0]	1 oz	0	0
Brazil nuts	[0]	1.75 oz	0	0
Breton wheat crackers	67	6 crackers	14	10
Broad beans	79	½ cup	11	9
Broccoli, raw	[0]	1 cup	0	0
Broken rice, white, cooked	86	1 cup	43	37
Brown rice, cooked	50	1 cup	33	16
Buckwheat	54	¾ cup	30	16
Bulgur, cooked 20 min	48	¾ cup	26	12
Bun, hamburger	61	1.5 oz	22	13
Butter beans, canned	31	⅔ cup	20	6
C				
Cabbage, raw	[0]	1 cup	0	0
Cactus Nectar, Organic Agave, light, 90% fructose (Western Commerce)	11	1 Tbsp	8	1
Cactus Nectar, Organic Agave, light, 97% fructose (Western Commerce)	10	1 Tbsp	8	1
Cantaloupe, fresh	65	4 oz	6	4
Cappellini pasta, cooked	45	1½ cups	45	20
Carrot juice, fresh	43	8 oz	23	10
Carrots, peeled, cooked	49	½ cup	5	2
Carrots, raw	47	1 medium	6	3
Cashew nuts, salted	22	1.75 oz	13	3
Cauliflower, raw	[0]	¾ cup	0	0
Celery, raw	[0]	2 stalks	0	0
Cheese	[0]	4 oz	0	0

[0] indicates that the food has so little carbohydrate that the GI value cannot be tested. The GL, therefore, is 0.

FOOD	GI Value	Nominal Serving Size	Net Carb per Serving	GL per Serving
Cherries, fresh	22	18	12	3
Chicken nuggets, frozen	46	4 oz	16	7
Chickpeas, canned	42	⅔ cup	22	9
Chickpeas, dried, cooked	28	⅔ cup	30	8
Chocolate cake made from mix with chocolate frosting	38	4 oz	52	20
Chocolate milk, low-fat	34	8 oz	26	9
Chocolate mousse, 2% fat	31	½ cup	22	7
Chocolate powder, dissolved in water	55	8 oz	16	9
Chocolate pudding, made from powder and whole milk	47	½ cup	24	11
Choice DM™, nutritional support product, vanilla (Mead Johnson)	23	8 oz	24	6
Clif® bar (cookies & cream)	101	2.4 oz	34	34
Coca Cola®, soft drink	53	8 oz	26	14
Cocoa Puffs™, breakfast cereal	77	1 cup	26	20
Complete™, breakfast cereal	48	1 cup	21	10
Condensed milk, sweetened	61	2½ Tbsps	27	17
Converted rice, long-grain, cooked 20-30 min, Uncle Ben's®	50	1 cup	36	18
Converted rice, white, cooked 20-30 min, Uncle Ben's®	38	1 cup	36	14
Corn Flakes™, breakfast cereal	92	1 cup	26	24
Corn Flakes™, Honey Crunch, breakfast cereal	72	¾ cup	25	18
Corn pasta, gluten-free	78	1¼ cups	42	32
Corn Pops™, breakfast cereal	80	1 cup	26	21
Corn Thins, puffed corn cakes, gluten-free	87	1 oz	20	18
Corn, sweet, cooked	60	½ cup	18	11
Cornmeal, cooked 2 min	68	1 cup	13	9
Couscous, cooked 5 min	65	¾ cup	35	23

[0] indicates that the food has so little carbohydrate that the GI value cannot be tested. The GL, therefore, is 0.

FOOD	GI Value	Nominal Serving Size	Net Carb per Serving	GL per Serving
Cranberry juice cocktail	52	8 oz	31	16
Crispix™, breakfast cereal	87	1 cup	25	22
Croissant, medium	67	2 oz	26	17
Cucumber, raw	[0]	¾ cup	0	0
Cupcake, strawberry-iced, small	73	1.5 oz	26	19
Custard apple, raw, flesh only	54	4 oz	19	10
Custard, homemade	43	½ cup	26	11
Custard, prepared from powder with whole milk, instant	35	½ cup	26	9
D				
Dates, dried	50	7	40	20
Desiree potato, peeled, cooked	101	5 oz	17	17
Doughnut, cake type	76	1.75 oz	23	17
E				
Eggs, large	[0]	2	0	0
Enercal Plus™ (Wyeth-Ayerst)	61	8 oz	40	24
English Muffin™ bread (Natural Ovens)	77	1 oz	14	11
Ensure™, vanilla drink	48	8 oz	34	16
Ensure™ bar, chocolate fudge brownie	43	1.4 oz	20	8
Ensure Plus™, vanilla drink	40	8 oz	47	19
Ensure Pudding™, old-fashioned vanilla	36	4 oz	26	9
F				
Fanta®, orange soft drink	68	8 oz	34	23
Fettuccine, egg, cooked	32	1½ cups	46	15
Figs, dried	61	3	26	16
Fish	[0]	4 oz	0	0
Fish sticks	38	3.5 oz	19	7
Flan/crème caramel	65	½ cup	73	47
French baguette, white, plain	95	1 oz	15	15

[0] indicates that the food has so little carbohydrate that the GI value cannot be tested. The GL, therefore, is 0.

FOOD	GI Value	Nominal Serving Size	Net Carb per Serving	GL per Serving
French fries, frozen, reheated in microwave	75	30 pcs	29	22
French green beans, cooked	[0]	½ cup	0	0
French vanilla cake made from mix, with vanilla frosting	42	4 oz	58	24
French vanilla ice cream, premium, 16% fat	38	½ cup	14	5
Froot Loops™, breakfast cereal	69	1 cup	26	18
Frosted Flakes™, breakfast cereal	55	1 cup	26	15
Fructose, pure	19	1 Tbsp	10	2
Fruit cocktail, canned, light syrup	55	½ cup	16	9
Fruit leather	61	2 pcs	24	15
G				
Gatorade™ (orange) sports drink	89	8 oz	15	13
Gin	[0]	1 oz	0	0
Glucerna™, vanilla (Abbott)	31	8 oz	23	7
Glucose (dextrose)	99	1 Tbsp	10	10
Glucose tablets	102	3 pcs	15	15
Gluten-free corn pasta	78	1½ cups	42	32
Gluten-free multigrain bread	79	1 oz	13	10
Gluten-free rice and corn pasta	76	1½ cups	49	37
Gluten-free spaghetti, rice and split pea, canned in tomato sauce	68	8 oz	27	19
Gluten-free split pea and soy pasta shells	29	1½ cups	31	9
Gluten-free white bread, sliced	80	1 oz	15	12
Glutinous (sticky) rice, white, cooked	92	⅔ cup	48	44
Gnocchi	68	6 oz	48	33
Grapefruit, fresh, medium	25	1 half	11	3
Grapefruit juice, unsweetened	48	8 oz	20	9
Grape-Nuts® (Post), breakfast cereal	75	¼ cup	21	16

[0] indicates that the food has so little carbohydrate that the GI value cannot be tested. The GL, therefore, is 0.

FOOD	GI Value	Nominal Serving Size	Net Carb per Serving	GL per Serving
Grapes, black, fresh	59	¾ cup	18	11
Grapes, green, fresh	46	¾ cup	18	8
Green peas	48	⅓ cup	7	3
Green pea soup, canned	66	8 oz	41	27
H				
Hamburger bun	61	1.5 oz	22	13
Happiness™ (cinnamon, raisin, pecan bread) (Natural Ovens)	63	1 oz	14	9
Hazelnuts	[0]	1.75 oz	0	0
Healthy Choice™ Hearty 100% Whole Grain	62	1 oz	14	9
Healthy Choice™ Hearty 7-Grain	55	1 oz	14	8
Heary Oatmeal cookies, FIFTY50	30	4 cookies	20	6
Honey	55	1 Tbsp	18	10
Hot cereal, apple & cinnamon, dry (Con Agra)	37	1.2 oz	22	8
Hot cereal, unflavored, dry (Con Agra)	25	1.2 oz	19	5
Hunger Filler™, whole-grain bread (Natural Ovens)	59	1 oz	13	7
I				
Ice cream, low-fat, vanilla, "light"	50	½ cup	9	5
Ice cream, premium, French vanilla, 16% fat	38	½ cup	14	5
Ice cream, premium, "ultra chocolate," 15% fat	37	½ cup	14	5
Ice cream, regular fat	61	½ cup	20	12
Instant potato, mashed	97	¾ cup	20	17
Instant rice, white, cooked 6 min	87	¾ cup	42	36
Ironman PR® bar, chocolate	39	2.3 oz	26	10

[0] indicates that the food has so little carbohydrate that the GI value cannot be tested. The GL, therefore, is 0.

FOOD	GI Value	Nominal Serving Size	Net Carb per Serving	GL per Serving
J				
Jam, apricot fruit spread, reduced sugar	55	1½ Tbsps	13	7
Jam, strawberry	51	1½ Tbsps	20	10
Jasmine rice, white, cooked	109	1 cup	42	46
Jelly beans	78	10 large	28	22
K				
Kaiser roll	73	1 half	16	12
Kavli™ Norwegian crispbread	71	5 pcs	16	12
Kidney beans, canned	52	⅔ cup	17	9
Kidney beans, cooked	23	⅔ cup	25	6
Kiwi fruit	53	4 oz	12	7
Kudos® Whole Grain Bars, chocolate chip	62	1.8 oz	32	20
L				
Lactose, pure	46	1 Tbsp	10	5
Lamb	[0]	4 oz	0	0
Leafy vegetables (spinach, arugula, etc.), raw	[0]	1½ cups	0	0
L.E.A.N Fibergy™ bar, Harvest Oat	45	1.75 oz	29	13
L.E.A.N Life long Nutribar™, Chocolate Crunch	32	1.5 oz	19	6
L.E.A.N Life long Nutribar™, Peanut Crunch	30	1.5 oz	19	6
L.E.A.N Nutrimeal™, drink powder, Dutch Chocolate	26	8 oz	13	3
Lemonade, reconstituted	66	8 oz	20	13
Lentil soup, canned	44	9 oz	21	9
Lentils, brown, cooked	29	¾ cup	18	5
Lentils, green, cooked	30	¾ cup	17	5
Lentils, red, cooked	26	¾ cup	18	5

[0] indicates that the food has so little carbohydrate that the GI value cannot be tested. The GL, therefore, is 0.

FOOD	GI Value	Nominal Serving Size	Net Carb per Serving	GL per Serving
Lettuce	[0]	4 leaves	0	0
Life Savers®, peppermint candy	70	18 pcs	30	21
Light rye bread	68	1 oz	14	10
Lima beans, baby, frozen	32	¾ cup	30	10
Linguine pasta, thick, cooked	46	1½ cups	48	22
Linguine pasta, thin, cooked	52	1½ cups	45	23
Long-grain rice, cooked 10 min	61	1 cup	36	22
Lychees, canned in syrup, drained	79	4 oz	20	16
M				
M & M's®, peanut	33	15 pcs	17	6
Macadamia nuts	[0]	1.75 oz	0	0
Macaroni and cheese, made from mix	64	1 cup	51	32
Macaroni, cooked	47	1¼ cups	48	23
Maltose	105	1 Tbsp	10	11
Mango	51	4 oz	15	8
Maple syrup, pure Canadian	54	1 Tbsp	18	10
Marmalade, orange	48	1½ Tbsps	20	9
Mars Bar®	68	2 oz	40	27
Melba toast, Old London	70	6 pcs	23	16
METRx® bar (vanilla)	74	3.6 oz	50	37
Milk Arrowroot™ cookies	69	5	18	12
Millet, cooked	71	⅔ cup	36	25
Mini Wheats™, whole-wheat breakfast cereal	58	12 pcs	21	12
Mousse, butterscotch, 1.9% fat	36	1.75 oz	10	4
Mousse, chocolate, 2% fat	31	1.75 oz	11	3
Mousse, hazelnut, 2.4% fat	36	1.75 oz	10	4
Mousse, mango, 1.8% fat	33	1.75 oz	11	4
Mousse, mixed berry, 2.2% fat	36	1.75 oz	10	4
Mousse, strawberry, 2.3% fat	32	1.75 oz	10	3

[0] indicates that the food has so little carbohydrate that the GI value cannot be tested. The GL, therefore, is 0.

FOOD	GI Value	Nominal Serving Size	Net Carb per Serving	GL per Serving
Muesli bar containing dried fruit	61	1 oz	21	13
Muesli bread, made from mix in bread oven (Con Agra)	54	1 oz	12	7
Muesli, gluten-free, with low-fat milk	39	1 oz	19	7
Muesli, Swiss Formula	56	1 oz	16	9
Muesli, toasted	43	1 oz	17	7
Multi-Grain 9-Grain bread	43	1 oz	14	6
N				
Navy beans, canned	38	5 oz	31	12
Nesquik™, chocolate dissolved in low-fat milk, no-sugar-added	41	8 oz	11	5
Nesquik™, strawberry dissolved in low-fat milk, no-sugar-added	35	8 oz	12	4
New creamer potato, canned	65	5 oz	18	12
New creamer potato, unpeeled and cooked 20 min	78	5 oz	21	16
Noodles, instant "two-minute" (Maggi®)	46	1½ cups	40	19
Noodles, mung bean (Lungkow beanthread), dried, cooked	39	1½ cups	45	18
Noodles, rice, fresh, cooked	40	1½ cups	39	15
Nutella®, chocolate hazelnut spread	33	1 Tbsp	12	4
Nutrigrain™, breakfast cereal	66	1 cup	15	10
Nutty Natural™, whole-grain bread (Natural Ovens)	59	1 oz	12	7
O				
Oat bran, raw	55	2 Tbsp	5	3
Oatmeal, cooked 1 min	66	1 cup	26	17
Oatmeal cookies	55	4 small	21	12
Oatmeal cookies, Sugar-Free, FIFTY50	47	4 cookies	28	10

[0] indicates that the food has so little carbohydrate that the GI value cannot be tested. The GL, therefore, is 0.

FOOD	GI Value	Nominal Serving Size	Net Carb per Serving	GL per Serving
Orange juice, unsweetened, reconstituted	53	8 oz	18	9
Orange, fresh, medium	42	4 oz	11	5
P				
Pancakes, buckwheat, gluten-free, made from mix	102	2 4" pancakes	22	22
Pancakes, made from mix	67	2 4" pancakes	58	39
Papaya, fresh	59	4 oz	8	5
Parsnips	97	½ cup	12	12
Pastry	59	2 oz	26	15
Pea soup, canned	66	8 oz	41	27
Peach, canned in heavy syrup	58	½ cup	26	15
Peach, canned in light syrup	52	½ cup	18	9
Peach, fresh, large	42	4 oz	11	5
Peanuts	14	1.75 oz	6	1
Pear halves, canned in natural juice	43	½ cup	13	5
Pear, fresh	38	4 oz	11	4
Peas, green, frozen, cooked	48	½ cup	7	3
Pecans	[0]	1.75 oz	0	0
Pepper, fresh, green or red	[0]	3 oz	0	0
Pineapple, fresh	66	4 oz	10	6
Pineapple juice, unsweetened	46	8 oz	34	15
Pinto beans, canned	45	⅔ cup	22	10
Pinto beans, dried, cooked	39	¾ cup	26	10
Pita bread, white	57	1 oz	17	10
Pizza, cheese	60	1 slice	27	16
Pizza, Super Supreme, pan (11.4% fat)	36	1 slice	24	9
Pizza, Super Supreme, thin and crispy (13.2% fat)	30	1 slice	22	7
Plums, fresh	39	2 medium	12	5
Pop Tarts™, double chocolate	70	1.8 oz pastry	36	25

[0] indicates that the food has so little carbohydrate that the GI value cannot be tested. The GL, therefore, is 0.

FOOD	GI Value	Nominal Serving Size	Net Carb per Serving	GL per Serving
Popcorn, plain, cooked in microwave oven	72	1½ cups	11	8
Pork	[0]	4 oz	0	0
Potato chips, plain, salted	54	2 oz	21	11
Potato, baked	85	5 oz	30	26
Potato, microwaved	82	5 oz	33	27
Pound cake (Sara Lee)	54	2 oz	28	15
PowerBar® (chocolate)	57	2.3 oz	42	24
Premium soda crackers	74	5 crackers	17	12
Pretzels	83	1 oz	20	16
Prunes, pitted	29	6	33	10
Pudding, instant, chocolate, made with whole milk	47	½ cup	24	11
Pudding, instant, vanilla, made with whole milk	40	½ cup	24	10
Puffed crispbread	81	1 oz	19	15
Puffed rice cakes, white	82	3 cakes	21	17
Puffed Wheat, breakfast cereal	80	2 cups	21	17
Pumpernickel rye kernel bread	41	1 oz	12	5
Pumpkin	75	3 oz	4	3

R

FOOD	GI Value	Nominal Serving Size	Net Carb per Serving	GL per Serving
Raisin Bran™, breakfast cereal	61	½ cup	19	12
Raisins	64	½ cup	44	28
Ravioli, meat-filled, cooked	39	6.5 oz	38	15
Red wine	[0]	3.5 oz	0	0
Red-skinned potato, peeled and microwaved on high for 6–7.5 min	79	5 oz	18	14
Red-skinned potato, peeled, boiled 35 min	88	5 oz	18	16
Red-skinned potato, peeled, mashed	91	5 oz	20	18

[0] indicates that the food has so little carbohydrate that the GI value cannot be tested. The GL, therefore, is 0.

FOOD	GI Value	Nominal Serving Size	Net Carb per Serving	GL per Serving
Resource Diabetic™, nutritional support product, vanilla (Novartis)	34	8 oz	23	8
Rice and corn pasta, gluten-free	76	1½ cups	49	37
Rice bran, extruded	19	1 oz	14	3
Rice cakes, white	82	3 cakes	21	17
Rice Krispies™, breakfast cereal	82	1¼ cups	26	22
Rice Krispies Treat™ bar	63	1 oz	24	15
Rice noodles, fresh, cooked	40	1½ cups	39	15
Rice, parboiled	72	1 cup	36	26
Rice pasta, brown, cooked 16 min	92	1½ cups	38	35
Rice vermicelli	58	1½ cups	39	22
Rolled oats	42	1 cup	21	9
Roll-Ups®, processed fruit snack	99	1 oz	25	24
Roman (cranberry) beans, fresh, cooked	46	¾ cup	18	8
Russet, baked potato	85	5 oz	30	26
Rutabaga, fresh, cooked	72	5 oz	10	7
Rye bread	58	1 oz	14	8
Ryvita® crackers	69	3 crackers	16	11
S				
Salami	[0]	4 oz	0	0
Salmon	[0]	4 oz	0	0
Sausages, fried	28	3.5 oz	3	1
Scones, plain	92	1 oz	9	8
Sebago potato, peeled, cooked	87	5 oz	17	14
Seeded rye bread	55	1 oz	13	7
Semolina, cooked (dry)	55	⅓ cup	50	28
Shellfish (shrimp, crab, lobster, etc.)	[0]	4 oz	0	0
Sherry	[0]	2 oz	0	0
Shortbread cookies	64	1 oz	16	10

[0] indicates that the food has so little carbohydrate that the GI value cannot be tested. The GL, therefore, is 0.

FOOD	GI Value	Nominal Serving Size	Net Carb per Serving	GL per Serving
Shredded Wheat™, breakfast cereal	75	⅔ cup	20	15
Shredded Wheat™ biscuits	62	1 oz	18	11
Skim milk	32	8 oz	13	4
Skittles®	70	45 pcs	45	32
Smacks™, breakfast cereal	71	¾ cup	23	11
Smoothie, raspberry (ConAgra)	33	8 oz	41	14
Snack bar, Apple Cinnamon (ConAgra)	40	1.75 oz	29	12
Snack bar, Peanut Butter & Choc-Chip (ConAgra)	37	1.75 oz	27	10
Snickers® bar	68	2.2 oz	35	23
Soda crackers, Premium	74	5 crackers	17	12
Soft drink, Coca Cola®	53	8 oz	26	14
Soft drink, Fanta®, orange	68	8 oz	34	23
Sourdough rye	48	1 oz	12	6
Sourdough wheat	54	1 oz	14	8
Soy & Flaxseed bread (mix in bread oven) (ConAgra)	50	1 oz	10	5
Soybeans, canned	14	1 cup	6	1
Soybeans, dried, cooked	20	1 cup	6	1
Spaghetti, durum wheat, cooked 20 min	64	1½ cups	43	27
Spaghetti, gluten-free, rice and split pea, canned in tomato sauce	68	8 oz	27	19
Spaghetti, white, cooked 5 min	38	1½ cups	48	18
Spaghetti, whole wheat, cooked 5 min	32	1½ cups	44	14
Special K™, breakfast cereal	69	1 cup	21	14
Spirali pasta, durum wheat, al dente	43	1½ cups	44	19
Split pea and soy pasta shells, gluten-free	29	1½ cups	31	9
Split-pea soup	60	1 cup	27	16
Split peas, yellow, cooked 20 min	32	¾ cup	19	6

[0] indicates that the food has so little carbohydrate that the GI value cannot be tested. The GL, therefore, is 0.

FOOD	GI Value	Nominal Serving Size	Net Carb per Serving	GL per Serving
Sponge cake, plain	46	2 oz	36	17
Squash, raw	[0]	⅔ cup	0	0
Star pastina, white, cooked 5 min	38	1½ cups	48	18
Stay Trim™, whole-grain bread (Natural Ovens)	70	1 oz	15	10
Stoned Wheat Thins	67	14 crackers	17	12
Strawberries, fresh	40	4 oz	3	1
Strawberry jam	51	1½ Tbsps	20	10
Strawberry shortcake	42	2.2 oz	40	17
Stuffing, bread	74	1 oz	21	16
Sucrose	68	1 Tbsp	10	7
Super Supreme pizza, pan (11.4% fat)	36	1 slice	24	9
Super Supreme pizza, thin and crispy (13.2% fat)	30	1 slice	22	7
Sushi, salmon	48	3.5 oz	36	17
Sweet corn, whole kernel, canned, diet-pack, drained	46	1 cup	28	13
Sweet potato, cooked	44	5 oz	25	11

T

FOOD	GI Value	Nominal Serving Size	Net Carb per Serving	GL per Serving
Taco shells, baked	68	2 shells	12	8
Tapioca, cooked with milk	81	¾ cup	18	14
Tofu-based frozen dessert, chocolate with high-fructose (24%) corn syrup	115	1.75 oz	9	10
Tomato juice, canned, no added sugar	38	8 oz	9	4
Tomato soup	38	1 cup	17	6
Tortellini, cheese	50	6.5 oz	21	10
Tortilla chips, plain, salted	63	1.75 oz	26	17
Total™, breakfast cereal	76	¾ cup	22	17
Tuna	[0]	4 oz	0	0
Twix® Cookie Bar, caramel	44	2 cookies	39	17

[0] indicates that the food has so little carbohydrate that the GI value cannot be tested. The GL, therefore, is 0.

FOOD	GI Value	Nominal Serving Size	Net Carb per Serving	GL per Serving
U				
Ultra chocolate ice cream, premium, 15% fat	37	½ cup	14	5
Ultracal™ with fiber (Mead Johnson)	40	8 oz	29	12
V				
Vanilla cake made from mix, with vanilla frosting	42	4 oz	58	24
Vanilla pudding, instant, made with whole milk	40	½ cup	24	10
Vanilla wafers, creme-filled, FIFTY50	41	4 cookies	20	8
Vanilla wafers	77	6 cookies	18	14
Veal	[0]	4 oz	0	0
Vermicelli, white, cooked	35	1½ cups	44	16
W				
Waffles, Aunt Jemima®	76	1 4" waffle	13	10
Walnuts	[0]	1.75 oz	0	0
Water crackers	78	7 crackers	18	14
Watermelon, fresh	72	4 oz	6	4
Weet-Bix™, breakfast cereal	69	2 biscuits	17	12
Wheaties™, breakfast cereal	82	1 cup	21	17
Whiskey	[0]	1 oz	0	0
White bread	70	1 oz	14	10
White rice, instant, cooked 6 min	87	1 cup	42	36
White wine	[0]	3.5 oz	0	0
100% Whole Grain™ bread (Natural Ovens)	51	1 oz	13	7
Whole milk	31	8 oz	12	4
Whole-wheat bread	77	1 oz	12	9
Wonder™ white bread	80	1 oz	14	11

[0] indicates that the food has so little carbohydrate that the GI value cannot be tested. The GL, therefore, is 0.

FOOD	GI Value	Nominal Serving Size	Net Carb per Serving	GL per Serving
X				
Xylitol	8	1 Tbsp	10	1
Y				
Yam, peeled, cooked	37	5 oz	36	13
Yogurt, low-fat, wild strawberry	31	8 oz	34	11
Yogurt, low-fat, with fruit and artificial sweetener	14	8 oz	15	2
Yogurt, low-fat, with fruit and sugar	33	8 oz	35	12

[0] indicates that the food has so little carbohydrate that the GI value cannot be tested. The GL, therefore, is 0.

18

LOW TO HIGH GI VALUES

FOR THOSE WHO wish to choose a diet with the lowest GI values possible, we've created the following listing in order of GI values (i.e., from lowest to highest value). We've also divided the list into food categories, so that when you want to find a low-GI vegetable or fruit, for example, the information is at your fingertips. The categories are:

- bakery products
- beverages
- breads
- breakfast foods
- cookies
- crackers
- dairy products and alternatives
- fruits and fruit products
- grains
- infant formulas and baby foods

- legumes
- meal-replacement products
- mixed meals and convenience foods
- noodles
- pasta
- protein foods
- snack foods and candy
- soups
- special dietary products
- sugars
- vegetables

As we discuss in *The New Glucose Revolution*, it's not necessary to eat all of your carbohydrates from low-GI sources. If half of your carbohydrate choices have low GI values, you're doing well. If you also eat a low-GI food at each meal, you'll be reducing the GI values overall.

FOOD	LOW	INTERMEDIATE	HIGH

BAKERY PRODUCTS

Cakes

FOOD	LOW	INTERMEDIATE	HIGH
Banana	○		
Chocolate, with chocolate frosting	○		
Pound	○		
Sponge	○		
Vanilla	○		
Angel food		◑	
Flan		◑	

Muffins

FOOD	LOW	INTERMEDIATE	HIGH
Apple with sugar or artificial sweeteners	○		
Apple, oat, and raisin	○		
Banana, oat, and honey		◑	
Bran		◑	
Blueberry		◑	
Carrot		◑	
Oatmeal, made from mix, Quaker Oats		◑	
Cupcake, iced			●
Scone, plain			●

Pastries

FOOD	LOW	INTERMEDIATE	HIGH
Croissant		◑	
Doughnut, cake-type			●

BEVERAGES

Alcoholic

FOOD	LOW	INTERMEDIATE	HIGH
Beer	○		
Brandy	○		

FOOD	LOW	INTERMEDIATE	HIGH
Gin	○		
Sherry	○		
Whiskey	○		
Wine, red	○		
Wine, white	○		
Juices			
Apple, with sugar or artificial sweetener	○		
Carrot, fresh	○		
Grapefruit, unsweetened	○		
Pineapple, unsweetened	○		
Tomato, canned, no added sugar	○		
Smoothies and Shakes			
Raspberry	○		
Soy	○		
Soft drinks			
Coca-Cola®		◑	
Fanta®		◑	
Sports drinks			
Gatorade®			●

BREADS

	LOW	INTERMEDIATE	HIGH
Fruit			
Muesli, made from mix	○		
Happiness™, cinnamon, raisin, pecan		◑	
Gluten-free			
Fiber-enriched			●
White			●

FOOD	LOW	INTERMEDIATE	HIGH
Rye			
Pumpernickel	○		
Sourdough	○		
Cocktail		◑	
Light		◑	
Whole-wheat		◑	
Spelt			
Multigrain	○		
White			●
Wheat			
100% Whole Grain	○		
Soy & Linseed bread machine mix	○		
Flatbread, Indian		◑	
Hearty 7 Grain		◑	
Pita, plain		◑	
Bagel			●
Baguette			●
Bread stuffing			●
English Muffin			●
Flatbread, Middle Eastern			●
Italian			●
Lebanese, white			●
White, enriched			●
Whole-wheat			●

FOOD	LOW	INTERMEDIATE	HIGH

BREAKFAST FOODS

Breakfast cereal bars

Rice Krispies® Treat		◑	

Cooked cereals

Hot cereal, apple & cinnamon, ConAgra	○		
Old-fashioned oats	○		
Cream of Wheat™, regular, Nabisco		◑	
One Minute Oats, Quaker Oats		◑	
Quick Oats, Quaker Oats		◑	
Cream of Wheat™, instant, Nabisco			●
Oatmeal, instant			●

Grain products

Pancakes, prepared from mix	○		
Pancakes, buckwheat, gluten-free, made from mix			●
Waffles, Aunt Jemima®			●

Ready-to-eat cereals

All-Bran®, Kellogg's	○		
Complete™ Bran Flakes, Kellogg's	○		
Bran Buds™, Kellogg's		◑	
Bran Chex™, Kellogg's		◑	
Froot Loops™, Kellogg's		◑	
Frosted Flakes™, Kellogg's		◑	
Just Right™, Kellogg's		◑	
Life™, Quaker Oats		◑	
Nutrigrain™, Kellogg's		◑	
Oat bran, raw, Quaker Oats		◑	
Puffed Wheat, Quaker Oats		◑	

FOOD	LOW	INTERMEDIATE	HIGH
Raisin Bran™, Kellogg's		◑	
Special K™, Kellogg's		◑	
Bran Flakes™, Kellogg's			●
Cheerios™, General Mills			●
Corn Chex™, Kellogg's			●
Corn Flakes™, Kellogg's			●
Corn Pops™, Kellogg's			●
Grapenuts™, Post			●
Rice Krispies™, Kellogg's			●
Shredded Wheat™, Nabisco			●
Team™ Flakes, Nabisco			●
Total™			●
Weetabix™			●

COOKIES

FOOD	LOW	INTERMEDIATE	HIGH
Hearty Oatmeal, FIFTY50	○		
Oatmeal, Sugar-Free, FIFTY50	○		
Vanilla wafers, creme filled, FIFTY50	○		
Arrowroot		◑	
Digestives		◑	
Tea biscuits		◑	
Shortbread		◑	
Vanilla wafers			●

CRACKERS

FOOD	LOW	INTERMEDIATE	HIGH
Breton wheat		◑	
Melba Toast		◑	
Rye crispbread		◑	
Ryvita™		◑	
Stoned Wheat Thins		◑	

FOOD	LOW	INTERMEDIATE	HIGH
Water		◑	
Kavli™ Norwegian Crispbread			●
Premium soda (Saltines)			●
Rice cakes, puffed			●

DAIRY PRODUCTS AND ALTERNATIVES

Custard

Homemade	○		

Ice cream

Regular	○		

Milk

Low-fat, chocolate, with aspartame	○		
Low-fat, chocolate, with sugar	○		
Skim	○		
Whole	○		
Condensed, sweetened			●

Mousse

Butterscotch, low-fat, Nestlé	○		
Chocolate, low-fat, Nestlé	○		
French vanilla, low-fat, Nestlé	○		
Hazelnut, low-fat, Nestlé	○		
Mango, low-fat, Nestlé	○		
Mixed berry, low-fat, Nestlé	○		
Strawberry, low-fat, Nestlé	○		

Pudding

Instant, chocolate, made with milk	○		
Instant, vanilla, made with milk	○		

FOOD	LOW	INTERMEDIATE	HIGH
Soy milk			
Reduced fat	○		
Whole	○		
Soy yogurt			
Tofu-based frozen dessert, chocolate			●
Yogurt			
Low-fat, fruit, with aspartame	○		
Low-fat, fruit, with sugar	○		
Nonfat, French vanilla, with sugar	○		
Nonfat, strawberry, with sugar	○		

FRUIT AND FRUIT PRODUCTS

FOOD	LOW	INTERMEDIATE	HIGH
Apple, fresh	○		
Apricot, fresh	○		
Banana, fresh	○		
Cantaloupe, fresh	○		
Cherries, fresh	○		
Grapefruit, fresh	○		
Grapes, fresh	○		
Kiwi, fresh	○		
Mango, fresh	○		
Orange, fresh	○		
Peach, canned in natural juice	○		
Peach, fresh	○		
Pear, canned in pear juice	○		
Pear, fresh	○		
Plum, fresh	○		
Prunes, pitted	○		
Strawberries, fresh	○		
Strawberry jam	○		
Figs, dried		◐	

FOOD	LOW	INTERMEDIATE	HIGH
Fruit cocktail, canned		◑	
Papaya, fresh		◑	
Peach, canned in heavy syrup		◑	
Peach, canned in light syrup		◑	
Pineapple, fresh		◑	
Raisins/sultanas		◑	
Dates, dried			●
Lychee, canned in syrup, drained			●
Watermelon, fresh			●

GRAINS

FOOD	LOW	INTERMEDIATE	HIGH
Barley, cracked	○		
Barley, pearled	○		
Buckwheat	○		
Buckwheat groats	○		
Bulgur	○		
Corn, canned, no salt added	○		
Rice, brown	○		
Rice, Cajun Style, Uncle Ben's®	○		
Rice, Long Grain and Wild, Uncle Ben's®	○		
Rice, parboiled, converted, white, cooked 20–30 min, Uncle Ben's®	○		
Barley, rolled		◑	
Corn, fresh		◑	
Cornmeal		◑	
Couscous		◑	
Rice, arborio (risotto)		◑	
Rice, Basmati		◑	
Rice, Garden Style, Uncle Ben's®		◑	
Rice, parboiled, long-grain, cooked 10 minutes		◑	
Millet			●

FOOD	LOW	INTERMEDIATE	HIGH
Rice, sticky			●
Rice, parboiled			●
Tapioca boiled with milk			●

INFANT FORMULA AND BABY FOODS

Baby foods

Apple, apricot, and banana, baby cereal		◑	
Chicken and noodles with vegetables, strained		◑	
Corn and rice, baby		◑	
Oatmeal, creamed, baby		◑	
Rice pudding, baby		◑	

Infant formula

SMA, 20 cal./fl oz, Wyeth	○		
Nursoy, soy-based, milk-free, Wyeth		◑	

LEGUMES

Beans

Baked, canned	○		
Butter, dried and cooked	○		
Kidney, canned	○		
Lima, baby, frozen	○		
Mung, cooked	○		
Navy, dried and cooked	○		
Pinto, cooked	○		
Soy, canned	○		

Lentils

Green, dried and cooked	○		
Red, dried and cooked	○		

FOOD	LOW	INTERMEDIATE	HIGH

Peas

	LOW	INTERMEDIATE	HIGH
Black-eyed	○		
Chickpeas/garbanzo beans, canned	○		
Split, yellow, cooked	○		

MEAL-REPLACEMENT PRODUCTS

	LOW	INTERMEDIATE	HIGH
Designer chocolate, sugar-free, Worldwide Sport Nutrition low-carbohydrate products	○		
L.E.A.N Fibergy™ bar, Harvest Oat, Usana	○		
L.E.A.N (Life long) Nutribar™, Peanut Crunch, Usana	○		
L.E.A.N (Life long) Nutribar™, Chocolate Crunch, Usana	○		

MIXED MEALS AND CONVENIENCE FOODS

	LOW	INTERMEDIATE	HIGH
Chicken nuggets, frozen, reheated	○		
Fish fillet, reduced fat, breaded	○		
Fish sticks	○		
Greek lentil stew with a bread roll, homemade	○		
Lean Cuisine™, chicken with rice	○		
Pizza, Super Supreme, pan, Pizza Hut	○		
Pizza, Super Supreme, thin and crispy, Pizza Hut	○		
Pizza, Vegetarian Supreme, thin and crispy, Pizza Hut	○		
Spaghetti Bolognese	○		
Sushi, salmon	○		
Tortellini, cheese, Stouffer	○		
Tuna patty, reduced fat	○		
Cheese sandwich, white bread		◑	
Kugel		◑	
Macaroni and cheese, boxed, Kraft		◑	
Peanut-butter sandwich, white/whole-wheat bread		◑	
Pizza, cheese, Pillsbury		◑	

FOOD	LOW	INTERMEDIATE	HIGH
Spaghetti, gluten-free, canned in tomato sauce		◑	
Sushi, roasted sea algae, vinegar and rice		◑	
Taco shells, cornmeal-based, baked, El Paso		◑	
White bread and butter		◑	
Stir-fried vegetables with chicken and rice, homemade			●

NOODLES

FOOD	LOW	INTERMEDIATE	HIGH
Instant	○		
Mung bean, Lungkow beanthread	○		
Rice, fresh, cooked	○		
Rice, dried, cooked		◑	
Udon, plain, reheated 5 min		◑	

PASTA

FOOD	LOW	INTERMEDIATE	HIGH
Capellini	○		
Fettuccine, egg	○		
Gluten-free, cornstarch	○		
Linguine, thick, fresh, durum wheat, white	○		
Linguine, thin, fresh, durum wheat	○		
Macaroni, plain, cooked	○		
Ravioli	○		
Spaghetti, cooked 5 min	○		
Spaghetti, cooked 22 min	○		
Spaghetti, protein-enriched, cooked 7 min	○		
Spaghetti, whole wheat	○		
Spirali, cooked, durum wheat	○		
Star pastina, cooked 5 min	○		
Tortellini	○		
Vermicelli	○		
Gnocchi		◑	

FOOD	LOW	INTERMEDIATE	HIGH
Rice vermicelli		◐	
Spaghetti, cooked 10 min, Barilla		◐	
Corn, gluten-free			●
Rice and corn, gluten-free			●
Rice, brown, cooked 16 min			●

PROTEIN FOODS

	LOW	INTERMEDIATE	HIGH
Beef	○		
Cheese	○		
Cold cuts	○		
Eggs	○		
Fish	○		
Lamb	○		
Pork	○		
Sausages	○		
Shellfish (shrimp, crab, lobster, etc.)	○		
Veal	○		

SNACK FOODS and CANDY

Candy

	LOW	INTERMEDIATE	HIGH
Nougat	○		
Jelly beans			●
Life Savers®			●
Skittles®			●

Chips

	LOW	INTERMEDIATE	HIGH
Corn, plain, salted, Doritos™	○		
Potato, plain, salted	○		

Chocolate bars

	LOW	INTERMEDIATE	HIGH
Milk, Cadbury's	○		

FOOD	LOW	INTERMEDIATE	HIGH
Milk, Dove®, Mars	○		
Milk, Nestlé	○		
White, Milky Bar®	○		
Mars Bar®		◑	
Snickers Bar®		◑	

Chocolate candy

	LOW	INTERMEDIATE	HIGH
M & M's®, peanut	☉		

Chocolate spread

	LOW	INTERMEDIATE	HIGH
Nutella®, chocolate hazelnut spread	○		

Dried-fruit bars

	LOW	INTERMEDIATE	HIGH
Fruit Roll-Ups®			●

Nuts

	LOW	INTERMEDIATE	HIGH
Cashews	○		
Peanuts	○		
Pecans	○		

Popcorn

	LOW	INTERMEDIATE	HIGH
Plain, microwaved			●

Pretzels

	LOW	INTERMEDIATE	HIGH
Plain, salted			●

Snack bars

	LOW	INTERMEDIATE	HIGH
Apple Cinnamon, Con Agra	○		
Peanut Butter & Choc-Chip	○		
Twix® Cookie Bar, caramel	○		
Kudos Whole Grain Bars, chocolate chip		◑	

Sports bars

	LOW	INTERMEDIATE	HIGH
Ironman PR bar®, chocolate	○		

FOOD	LOW	INTERMEDIATE	HIGH
PowerBar®, chocolate		◐	

SOUPS

FOOD	LOW	INTERMEDIATE	HIGH
Lentil, canned	○		
Minestrone, canned, ready-to-serve	○		
Tomato, canned	○		
Black bean, canned		◐	
Green pea, canned		◐	
Split pea, canned		◐	

SPECIAL DIETARY PRODUCTS

FOOD	LOW	INTERMEDIATE	HIGH
Choice DM™, vanilla, Mead Johnson	○		
Ensure™, Abbott	○		
Ensure Plus™, vanilla, Abbott	○		
Ensure Pudding™, vanilla, Abbott	○		
Ensure™ bar, chocolate fudge brownie, Abbott	○		
Ensure™, vanilla, Abbott	○		
Glucerna™ bar, lemon crunch, Abbott	○		
Glucerna™ SR shake, vanilla, Abbott	○		
Glucerna™, vanilla, Abbott	○		
Resource Diabetic™, vanilla, Novartis	○		
Resource Plus, chocolate, Novartis	○		
Ultracal™ with fiber, Mead Johnson	○		
Enercal Plus™, Wyeth-Ayerst		◐	
Enrich Plus shake, vanilla, Ross		◐	

SUGARS

FOOD	LOW	INTERMEDIATE	HIGH
Blue Agave, Organic Agave Cactus Nectar, light, 90% fructose, Western Commerce	○		
Blue Agave, Organic Agave Cactus Nectar, light, 97% fructose, Western Commerce	○		
Fructose	○		

FOOD	LOW	INTERMEDIATE	HIGH
Lactose	○		
Honey		◑	
Sucrose		◑	
Glucose			●
Maltose			●

VEGETABLES

FOOD	LOW	INTERMEDIATE	HIGH
Artichokes	○		
Avocado	○		
Bok choy	○		
Broccoli	○		
Cabbage	○		
Carrots, peeled, cooked	○		
Cassava (yucca), cooked with salt	○		
Cauliflower	○		
Celery	○		
Corn, canned, no salt added	○		
Cucumber	○		
French beans (runner beans)	○		
Leafy greens	○		
Lettuce	○		
Peas, frozen, cooked	○		
Pepper	○		
Potato, sweet	○		
Squash	○		
Yam	○		
Beet		◑	
Corn, sweet, cooked		◑	
Potato, boiled/canned		◑	
Potato, new, canned		◑	
Taro		◑	

FOOD	LOW	INTERMEDIATE	HIGH
Broad beans			●
Parsnips			●
Potato, French fries, frozen and reheated			●
Potato, instant			●
Potato, mashed			●
Potato, microwaved			●
Potato, russet, baked			●
Pumpkin			●
Rutabaga			●

FOR MORE INFORMATION

To find a dietitian

The American Dietetic Association
120 S. Riverside Plaza
Suite 2000
Chicago, IL 60606
Phone: 1-800-877-1600
www.eatright.org

To order Natural Ovens bread

Natural Ovens Bakery
PO Box 730
Manitowoc, WI 54221-0730
Phone: 1-800-772-0730
www.naturalovens.com

To order FIFTY50 Foods or find your nearest retailer:

FIFTY50 Foods

PO Box 89
Mendham, NJ 07945
Phone: 1-973-543-7006
www.fifty50.com

Primary Care Physicians

If you think you need help with a weight problem, it's always a good idea to see your primary care physician for an evaluation.

Community Support Groups

Many communities offer support groups targeting people who are trying to lose weight. Your primary care physician or local hospital may be able to direct you to a support group best suited to your needs.

Diabetes Organizations

Extra weight can often make a diabetic condition worse. For more information about living with and controlling your diabetes, contact the following:

The American Diabetes Association
1701 North Beauregard Street
Alexandria, VA 22311
Phone: 1-800-DIABETES (1-800-342-2383)
http://www.diabetes.org/

Canadian Diabetes Association
National Office
15 Toronto Street, Suite 800
Toronto, ON M5C 2E3
Phone: 1-416-363-3373
1-800-BANTING (1-800-226-8464)
http://www.diabetes.ca/

GLYCEMIC INDEX TESTING

*I*F YOU ARE a food manufacturer, you may be interested in having the glycemic index value of some of your products tested on a fee-for-service basis. For more information, contact:

Sydney University Glycaemic Index Research Service (SUGiRS)
Department of Biochemistry
University of Sydney
NSW 2006 Australia
Fax: (61) (2) 9351-6022
E-mail: j.brandmiller@staff.usyd.edu.au

ACKNOWLEDGMENTS

We WOULD LIKE to thank Linda Rao, M.Ed., for her editorial work on the American edition.